FUNCTIONAL BANDAGING
Including Splints and Protective Dressings

FUNCTIONAL BANDAGING
Including Splints and Protective Dressings

Seymour W. Meyer, M.D., F.A.C.S., D-S

Director of Surgery
Deepdale General Hospital, Queens, N.Y.

Attending Surgeon
St. Johns Episcopal Hospital, Brooklyn, N.Y.

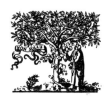

AMERICAN ELSEVIER PUBLISHING COMPANY, INC.

NEW YORK   1967

SOLE DISTRIBUTORS FOR GREAT BRITAIN
ELSEVIER PUBLISHING COMPANY, LTD.
Barking, Essex, England

SOLE DISTRIBUTORS FOR THE CONTINENT OF EUROPE
ELSEVIER PUBLISHING COMPANY
Amsterdam, The Netherlands

Library of Congress Catalog Card Number: 66-30438

To my wife, Beth,
and sons, Bobby and Ricky,
this work is affectionately
dedicated

PREFACE

The past twenty-five years have seen many advances in medicine and surgery. With so much interest focused on new surgical procedures as well as new techniques for treating fractures and other injuries, there has been an unfortunate neglect of a most important aspect, namely, the application of bandages and protective dressings.

The purpose of this book is twofold: one, to present a simple, logical method of bandaging which, once learned, should never be forgotten; and two, to review the basic techniques and materials for the application of a variety of protective dressings.

An unprecedented number of illustrations has been made to show the step-by-step application of the various bandages and surgical dressings. The reader sees the bandaging develop as though he were witnessing a motion picture. Each turn of bandage is carefully numbered. Nothing is left to the imagination.

This novel approach to a most vital subject, introduced by the author in a previous publication, has been modified to include many of the newer materials which have been developed in recent years.

This book should prove of value to physicians, medical students, nurses and nursing students, Army, Navy, and Air Corps medical personnel, and all others directly concerned with the care of the injured.

It is the hope of the author that this work will arouse a new interest in a sadly-neglected art.

S. W. MEYER

April 1967

ACKNOWLEDGMENTS

The author wishes to extend his thanks and appreciation to the following manufacturers of surgical materials and appliances for their kind cooperation in supplying photographs of some of their products referred to in the text.

Johnson & Johnson, New Brunswick, N. J.
Figs. 19, 20, 414, 520, 522, 527.

Zimmer Manufacturing Company, Warsaw, Indiana.
Figs. 9, 17, 471, 472, 474, 479, 480, 483, 484, 492, 493, 494, 497, 498, 499, 501, 502, 523, 524.

CONTENTS

Preface vii
Acknowledgments viii

UNIT ONE
Introduction

1. Simplicity in Bandaging 3
2. The Requirements of a Good Bandage 6
3. Definitions and Terminology 8
4. Materials used in Bandages, Splints, and Protective Dressings ... 17

UNIT TWO
Elementary Bandaging

5. The Basic Turns 27
6. Bandaging of Cylinders 29
7. Bandaging of Cones 33
8. Bandaging of Ovoids 39
9. The Figure-of-Eight Turns—Bandaging of Joints 43
10. Starting and Terminating of Bandages 48
11. Axioms of Good Functional Bandaging 54

UNIT THREE
Advanced Regional Bandaging

12. Introduction to Advanced Regional Bandaging 59
13. Bandages for the Upper Extremity 65
14. Bandages for the Lower Extremity 90
15. Bandages for the Head, Face, and Neck 108
16. Bandages for the Neck, Chest, and Axilla 117
17. Bandages for the Chest and Abdomen 122
18. Bandages for the Breasts 130
19. Bandages for the Arm, Chest, and Shoulder 136
20. Bandages for the Groin, Perineum, and Buttocks 147

UNIT FOUR
The Triangular Bandage

21. Preparation of the Triangle 155
22. Basic Principles and Techniques of Use 158
23. Regional Bandaging with the Triangle 161

UNIT FIVE

24. Adhesive Plaster Dressings and Taping 191

UNIT SIX
Splints

25. Basic Principles and Standard Splints 223
26. Emergency Splinting of Fractures 243

UNIT SEVEN

27. Plaster-of-Paris Dressings 253

UNIT EIGHT

28. Cosmetic Bandaging and Dressing 269

UNIT NINE

29. A practical Method of Presenting Bandaging 281

UNIT TEN

30. Bibliography 287
Index 290

UNIT ONE . . .

INTRODUCTION

"I dress it, God heals it."
Ambrose Paré

CONTENTS OF UNIT ONE

Introduction

Chapter 1

Simplicity in Bandaging

Chapter 2

The Requirements of a Good Bandage:
Functional Bandaging

Chapter 3

Definitions and Terminology

Chapter 4

Materials Used in Bandages, Splints,
and Protective Dressings

1

Simplicity in Bandaging

A method will be presented simplifying the entire scope of bandaging, both from the viewpoint of learning the techniques as well as the practical application of bandages to various parts of the body.

Instead of memorizing a wide variety of individual bandages for each part of the body, the bandager need visualize the body as being composed of only three basic geometric structures: (See Fig. 1, and Tables I and II.)

1. *Cylinders:* neck, trunk, wrists, lower legs, fingers, and toes.

2. *Truncated cones:* forearms, arms, legs, thighs, and feet.

3. *Ovoids:* head, finger tips, and tips of toes.

By acquiring skill in the application of dressings to these simple units of structure, the bandager is able to move freely from one part of the body to another, applying two hundred or more regional bandages with the utmost simplicity, dexterity, and ease.

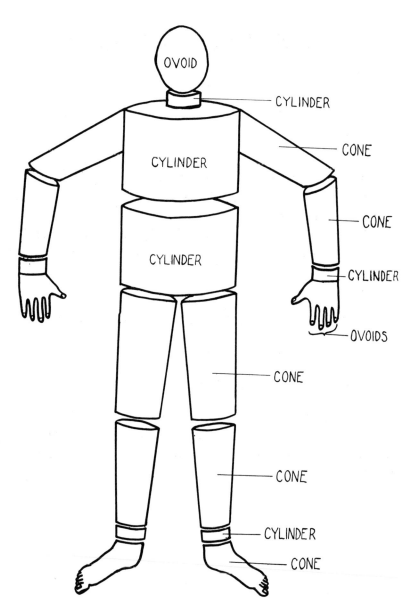

Figure 1

TABLE I

Geometric Configuration of the Body

Cylinders	Cones	Ovoids
Neck	Arms	Head
Thorax	Forearms	Finger tips
Abdomen	Thighs	Toe tips
Wrists	Legs	(Amputation
Fingers	Feet	stumps)
Lower legs		
(above ankles)		
Toes		

TABLE II

Alphabetical Index of Geometric Configurations

Part of Body	Geometric Configurations
Abdomen	cylinder
Arm	cone
Foot	cone
Finger	cylinder
Finger tip	ovoid
Forearm	cone
Head	ovoid
Leg	cone
Lower leg (above ankle)	cylinder
Neck	cylinder
Thigh	cone
Thorax	cylinder
Toe	cylinder
Toe tip	ovoid
Wrist	cylinder

2

The Requirements of a Good Bandage: Functional Bandaging

Functional Bandaging—Respect for Living Tissues

Much has been written of the surgeon's "respect for living tissues" in operative procedures. This delicate handling of tissues must also be applied in the art of bandaging. One must not inadvertently add further injury or trauma to tissues already damaged.

The bandager, at all times, must bear in mind that he is dealing with vital tissues and organs. This requires care as to the exact site and extent of injury, the condition of the circulation, the presence or absence of swelling, the degree of pressure, the relation of the injured parts to joints, the possibility of infection, and last, but far from least, the comfort of the patient. This means that the bandager must think in terms of vessels, of nerves, of muscles, of skin and its appendages (hair, nails, and glands), and to keep in mind the restoration and preservation of normal function.

This concept of *Functional Bandaging,* with its respect for living tissues, should be kept in mind by physician, nurse, armed forces personnel, trained bandager, and all others associated with the care of the injured patient.

Purposes and Functions of Bandages

Bandages are used for a variety of purposes, the most important of which are:
1. To protect injured areas
2. To hold dressings and splints in place
3. To exert pressure
4. To support parts of the body
5. To restrict or limit motion
6. To deplete a part of the body of its blood supply

6

The Good Bandage

From a practical viewpoint, the bandage which serves its function in relation to the underlying pathological process for which it is applied, may be considered a good bandage. The good bandager, not content to achieve only this goal, will regard his work as did Hippocrates, who informed us nearly 500 years B.C. that: "There are two views to bandaging; that which regards it while doing, and that which regards it when done. It should be done quickly, without pain, with ease, and with elegance; quickly, by despatching the work; without pain, by being readily done; with ease, by being prepared for everything; and with elegance, so that it may be agreeable to the sight." Thus, we may consider two phases of bandaging.

1. *The Technique of Bandaging with Respect to:*
   (a) Ease of performance
   (b) Speed
   (c) Use of available material
   (d) Adaptability to the individual case at hand

2. *The Completed Dressing or Bandage with Respect to:*
   (a) The patient
   (b) The bandager

To achieve perfection in the technique of bandaging, one must have a clear and comprehensive view of the various methods and materials used.

From the patient's viewpoint, the completed bandage must serve its primary purpose of protection, support, and promotion of repair. At the same time, the patient should enjoy the maximum comfort possible, without interference with the basic functions of the bandage.

For the bandager, the completed dressing or bandage acts as a spokesman. A well-applied bandage leads to earlier and better healing of the part, requires less frequent change, and in general reflects well upon the bandager. A neat-looking, well-balanced bandage indicates a certain dexterity, care, and pride of the bandager in his work, and thereby gains the confidence of the patient.

In the attempt to satisfy successfully both phases of bandaging, one must not sacrifice one completely for the other. Thus, to take twenty minutes to make an aesthetically-perfect bandage, which should ordinarily take three to five minutes, is not the end for which one is to strive.

A balance must be achieved between the ease of performance, speed, and adaptability to the individual case, and the production of a bandage which serves its primary purpose, is comfortable to the patient, and is neat in appearance.

3

Definitions and Terminology

A good bandager is thoroughly familiar with: (a) all of the terminology which surrounds his art, and (b) the materials which he employs in the practice of his art.

This chapter takes up the language of bandaging; the following one will describe the materials employed.

GLOSSARY OF TERMS

Bandage (French, *bande,* a strip)—Bandages are usually strips of muslin or other materials, of varying lengths and widths, used in surgery for the purpose of protecting or compressing a part, or for the retention of dressings or medications upon wounds.

Bandager—One skilled in the application of bandages.

Bandagist—A maker of trusses, bandages, and other surgical appliances to be worn upon the person.

Binder—A wide bandage about the abdomen, worn by patients after abdominal operations, or by women after childbirth, to support the abdominal walls. The *tailed bandages,* later described, are occasionally referred to as binders.

Compound Bandage—A bandage which consists of two or more pieces of material. For example, see *roller, double,* and *tailed bandages.*

Cravat Bandages—These are bandages prepared by folding a rectangular or triangular piece of material several times until a narrow strip is obtained, resembling a cravat. This is then used to bandage a part. (See *Handkerchief Bandages.*)

Dislocation—The displacement of one or more bones of a joint, so that the articular surfaces are not in normal apposition.

Fracture—A break in the continuity of a bone, either partial or complete. There are two main types:

1. *Simple:* A fracture in which the fragments of bone have not broken through the skin.

2. *Compound:* A fracture in which there is a communication between the fractured surfaces of bone and the surface of the body. Thus, it may be made by the sharp end of a fractured bone which penetrates the skin, or by a bullet, or other firm metallic object which passes in from the outside, and fractures the bone.

Figure 2

Handkerchief Bandages—These are prepared from a large handkerchief, or square or rectangular-shaped piece of material, which is folded to any desired width. (See Fig. 2.) When folded to a narrow width, a

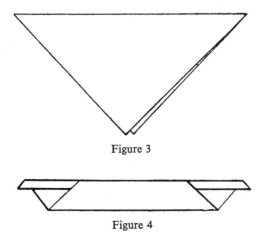

Figure 3

Figure 4

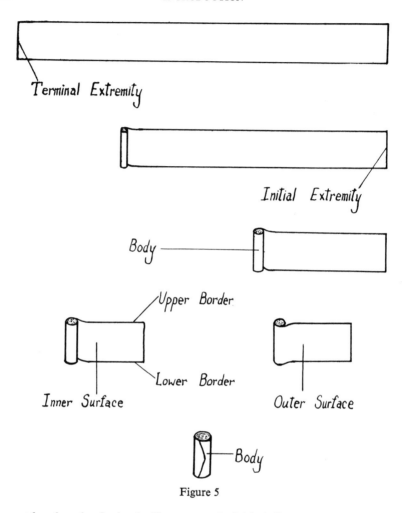

Figure 5

cravat bandage is obtained. If a square is folded diagonally, two triangles are obtained. The triangle may also be folded to a cravat. (See Figs. 3, 4.)

Immobilization Bandage—A form of bandage which is applied for the purpose of keeping a part in a particular position, until the injured or diseased tissues have had an opportunity to heal. Adhesive plaster and plaster-of-Paris dressings are included in this group.

Immovable Bandages—Same as *immobilization bandages.*

Movable Bandage—In contrast to immobilization bandages, this is a form of bandage which is applied merely to cover an injured surface; however, it does not immobilize a part. This type includes the commonly-used gauze and linen bandages.

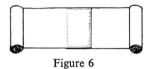

Figure 6

Pronation—A position of the hand in which the palm faces downward.

Roller Bandage (roller)—A strip of muslin, or other material, rolled into a cylindrical form. The length and width are variable. When referring to the *roller bandage,* one implies the *single roller,* to be distinguished from the *double roller,* later described. The single roller consists of seven parts:

1. *Initial Extremity:* The free end of the roller; that is, the end which unwinds.

2. *Terminal Extremity:* The end of the roller which is in the center of the cylinder. It is the last part of the roller to be unwound.

3 and 4. *Upper and Lower Borders:* The borders of the cylinder, which are determined by the positions these occupy when the patient stands erect.

5 and 6. *Inner and Outer Surfaces:* The surfaces of the material with respect to their relation to the center of the cylinder.

7. *Body:* This refers to the whole of the cylinder and includes all of the components. (See Fig. 5.)

Roller Bandage (double)—This consists of two single rollers, the initial extremities of which have been pinned or sewed together. (See Fig. 6.)

Scultetus Bandage—This is a many-tailed bandage which is prepared by sewing several strips of roller bandage together, each overlapping the next, in a shingle fashion. These are attached along the middle quarter of the strips, leaving the ends free. (See Fig. 7.)

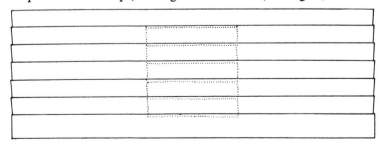

Figure 7

Simple Bandage—A bandage which consists of one piece of material. Same as the *roller bandage*.

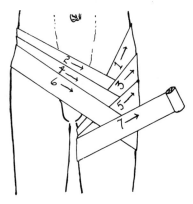

Figure 8

Spica Bandage—A bandage in which the turns resemble the arrangement of the husks of an ear of corn. It consists of two sets of turns, alternating with one another, and coming into contact at the area where it is intended to apply pressure or retain a dressing. (See *Spica of Groin,* Fig. 8.)

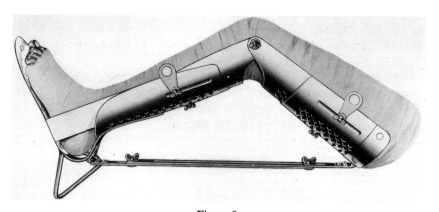

Figure 9

Splint—A piece of wood, metal, or other material employed for keeping the ends of a fractured bone or other movable parts in a state of rest. (See Fig. 9.)

Sprain—A wrenching or twisting of a joint, resulting in a stretching of the ligaments. Over small areas, there is actual tearing of the fibers. Often, the tendons and their sheaths may be injured.

Strain—An overstretching of a muscle which results in a parting of individual fibers of that muscle. Rarely is there actual rupture of large muscle bundles.

Subluxation—The displacement of one or more bones of a joint, of such a nature that the opposed joint surfaces are still partly in contact.

Supination—A position of the hand in which the palm faces upward.

Tailed Bandages—These are a group of bandages characterized by the presence of varying numbers of tails or ends. Each bandage consists of a body and three or more ends. The name of the bandage is determined by the number of tails or ends and the relative position of the components of the bandage. Tailed bandages are occasionally referred to as *binders*. The various types of tailed bandages are:

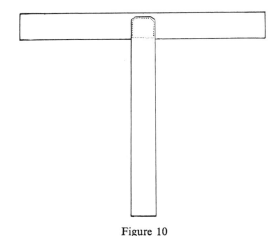

Figure 10

1. *The T-Bandage:* Consists of two strips of material sewed at right angles to each other to form a simple *T*. (See Fig. 10.)

2. *The Double-T-Bandage:* Consists of three strips of material, two attached at varying angles to the third, to form a double *T*. (See Fig. 11.)

This may also be formed by simply splitting the vertical piece of a simple *T-bandage*. (See Fig. 12.)

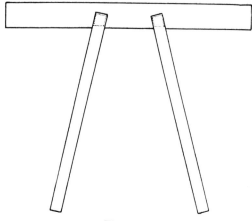

Figure 11

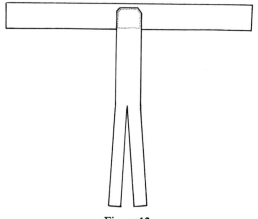

Figure 12

3. *The Four-tailed Bandage:* Consists of a piece of material cut so as to produce two tails at each end. (See Fig. 13.)

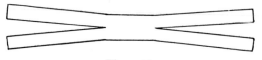

Figure 13

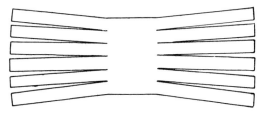

Figure 14

4. *The Many-tailed Bandage:* Consists of a piece of material cut toward the center so as to make three or more tails on either end. (See Fig. 14.) This is similar to the Scultetus bandage.

Taping—This refers to the immobilization of a part by the application of an adhesive plaster dressing.

Triangle Bandage—A triangular-shaped piece of material used, especially in emergencies, for bandaging various parts of the body. It is employed in its full size or is folded to any desired width. (See *Handkerchief Bandages* and Unit IV, *The Triangular Bandage.*)

4

Materials Used in Bandages, Splints, and Protective Dressings

Introduction

A knowledge of the materials which are available for use is as important to the surgical bandager as are the various techniques employed in the application of the bandages.

Where firm support must be given to an extremity, a moderately heavy and strong fabric must be used. Where a bandage is used merely to hold a light dressing in place, a thin, light, comfortable material should be employed. Where economy requires repeated use of supportive dressings, durable and washable fabrics should be used. The bandager who is thoroughly familiar with the types of materials available for his use, as well as the correct indications for same, will accomplish several desirable aims which include:

1. A bandage which serves its function well, thereby aiding in the maximum healing and repair of tissues.

2. A bandage which does not require too frequent change, leading to greater economy.

3. A bandage which is both neat and comfortable for the patient.

4. A bandage which further recommends and identifies the bandager as one who is both thorough and dependable in his attention to detail.

Classification of Materials

A wide variety of materials has been employed for the production of bandages and surgical dressings. Many of these have stood the test of time and practice and are still widely used. In recent years, however, many new materials have been produced which have done much to improve the ease and efficiency of bandaging and have added considerably to the comfort of the patient. Description and sources of these will be presented so that the reader may have the advantages of their use.

For convenience, these materials have been alphabetically arranged as follows:

Absorbent Cotton—A form of cotton which is treated in such manner as to remove its oils and waxes, thereby rendering it capable of absorbing fluids. Absorbent cotten is often used for cleansing, applying medications, as a padding for splints, and as a filler for dressings in between layers of gauze. (See Fig. 15.) Absorbent cotton must not be allowed to come directly into contact with the wound, since it tends to adhere to the edges of the wound, making its removal painful to the patient.

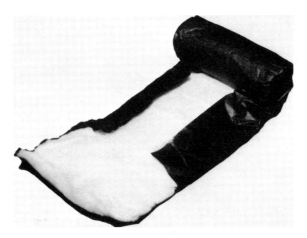

Figure 15

Adhesive Plaster—A material prepared by spreading a mixture of zinc oxide, waxes, resins, and rubber onto one surface of a firm cloth. When applied to a surface, this material has the ability to adhere firmly, and thus it is used to provide pressure, or support, and to hold dressings in place. Numerous variations in formula and substitutes for the conventional adhesive plaster have been produced in recent years. (For a more detailed discussion, see UNIT V, *Adhesive Plaster Dressings.*)

Cellulose—Prepared from wood pulp, cellulose consists of many layers of thin paper sheets which are bleached to a pure white. It has a soft texture, is very absorbent, and therefore is most often used as a substitute for cotton in various gauze-covered dressings. For copiously-discharging wounds, it is preferable to cotton since it is more economical.

Compression Bandages—These are made of specially prepared materials, used for maintenance of even pressure over various parts of the body, and for limitation of motion at joints. (See *Webbing,* in this chapter.)

Cotton Wadding—Nonabsorbent cotton which is prepared in sheet form and then rolled into bandages of various lengths and widths. It is used primarily as a protective material over delicate parts, as a padding under splints, and as a protective covering where skin surfaces come into contact under adhesive plaster or other types of dressings.

Crinoline—A loosely woven gauze material which is made stiff by treating it with starch. The main use for crinoline is in the preparation of plaster-of-Paris roller bandages, the loose mesh of the material serving to retain the plaster in place.

Dressing Combines—Large combination dressings used for the protection of operative wounds. They are so constructed as to absorb drainage from these wounds. A layer of absorbent cotton, backed by a layer of nonabsorbent cotton, is enclosed in gauze. The absorbent cotton side is applied over the wound. Cellulose may be used as a substitute for the absorbent cotton. The fluid-repellent, nonabsorbent cotton serves to confine the drainage to the dressing, thereby protecting the clothing and surrounding areas. (See Fig. 16.)

Felt—An unwoven fabric made of wool, or wool and hair, compressed by pressure and heat. It is prepared in various thicknesses and is used for padding in splints and casts. (See Fig. 17.)

Flannel—A soft, pliable, and resistant material, made of wool. It is cut from wide rolls into desired widths and then rolled by hand. Flannel is of value where protection, softness, and elasticity are desired. It adapts itself readily to a part, with very little tendency to become displaced. It maintains the temperature of a part and readily absorbs fluid. The main disadvantage of this material is that it may uselessly heat a part and irritate the skin by retaining moisture.

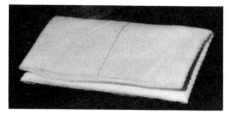

Figure 16

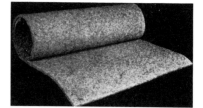

Figure 17

Foam Rubber—Prepared in sheets of varying thickness, of a highly porous rubber, this material is used for protection of bony surfaces exposed to pressure. A recent substitute for foam rubber has been urethane foam (Reston®), prepared in sheets, with a synthetic adhesive on one side. Designed primarily for the prevention of bed sores and decubitus ulcers, this material can also be used to protect pressure points in any areas.

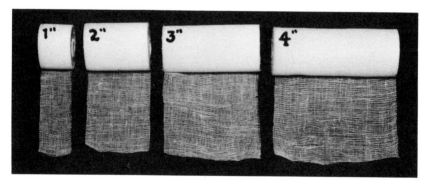

Figure 18

Gauze—Probably the most widely used of all surgical dressing materials. Gauze is a light, cool, and loosely woven absorbent material. It usually comes in rollers of various widths, ready for use. (See Fig. 18.) It is also prepared in wide rolls which may be cut to any desired width. The material is extremely pliable, making it valuable for the retention of dressings and splints. Gauze is graded according to its mesh, that is, the number of threads running lengthwise, and the number running crosswise, in a square inch of material. (See Fig. 19.) Where gauze is used merely as a covering, as in the *dressing combines,* the looser mesh is used. Where extra strength and protection are required, the closer meshed gauze is used.

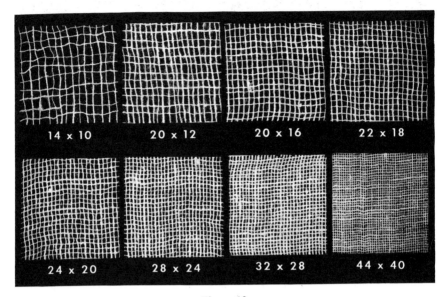

Figure 19

A new type of elastic gauze has been devised which has contributed much to bandaging. Produced commercially in roller bandages, and known as Kling®, it has two main advantages: easy conformity to body contour, and moderate stretch, allowing it to retain its position on parts that are subject to motion, i.e., extremities and joints.

Gauze Sponges—Pieces of gauze, folded to various sizes and thicknesses, used to cover and protect wounds. They are also used to absorb blood, pus, or other fluids during operations. Gauze sponges may be applied firmly to wounds for affording pressure in the control of hemorrhage. (See Fig. 20.)

Muslin—A tightly woven, unbleached material, heavier and stronger than gauze (50 × 60 mesh), but not as pliable. Muslin is employed where support and pressure, rather than elasticity, are needed. It is of value in the learning of bandaging since it is not pliable, and thus each turn must be perfectly applied, otherwise the bandage does not lie neatly. Muslin is used for the preparation of triangular and cravat bandages. Because of its strength, it is often used for maintenance of traction in the application of various emergency splints. Muslin also has the added advantage that it can be washed and used repeatedly.

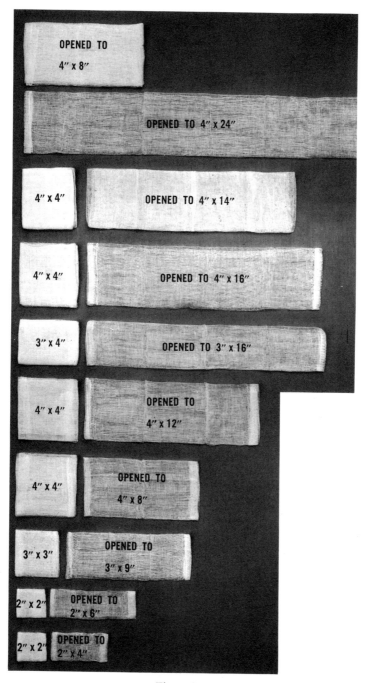

Figure 20

Nonabsorbent Cotton—A form of cotton in which the natural oils and waxes are retained, making it fluid repellent. Thus it is useful as a backing material for dressings which are applied over draining wounds. It protects the surrounding areas and clothing from the fluids. Nonabsorbent cotton is used in the preparation of cotton wadding and dressing combines, described previously.

Nonadherent Dressings—Since practically every surgical wound has some seepage of blood or serum, the conventional gauze dressing tends to become adherent to the skin edges. Removal of these pulls on the tissues and produces pain. This is particularly true in large open wounds, such as burns and skin graft sites. To eliminate this painful removal of dressings, special dressings have been devised with nonadherent inner surfaces which are applied directly to the wound. A commonly-used preparation, Telfa®, has an inner layer of plastic film, perforated with many small holes to allow seepage of blood or serum to flow into an outer layer of absorbent material. Microdon® surgical dressing is a complete unit for dressing a surgical wound, consisting of an inner nonadherent surface, an adjacent absorbent layer, and an adhesive to hold the entire dressing in place. Gauze impregnated with petrolatum, Vaseline Gauze®, has been used extensively as a nonadherent dressing, particularly in burns. Furacin Gauze® is a similar product which has an antiseptic incorporated into the material. Adaptic® is a nonadhering dressing consisting of a fabric of viscose filaments impregnated with a bland emulsion.

Rubber—Bandages are prepared of rubber in various lengths and widths. These are employed for the exertion of pressure and restriction of circulation to a part. (See *Webbing*.)

Stockinet—A tubular covering which is slipped over the arm, leg, or body, before the application of a plaster of Paris cast. The material is unbleached, nonabsorbent, and highly stretchable and serves to protect the skin and make the cast more comfortable. (See Fig. 21.)

Webbing—A material woven of long-fiber cotton threads. A special weave makes it elastic, so that it may be stretched to almost twice its length. It is used for even exertion of pressure and limitation of motion at joints. Webbing is commercially prepared in rollers of various widths. To increase and maintain the elasticity of webbing, threads of rubber are incorporated into the weaving. These are commonly referred to as Ace Bandages®. (See Fig. 22.) Recently, the rubber in these bandages has been replaced by a polyurethane plastic synthetic fiber which acts like rubber, but is lighter, cooler, softer, and stronger.

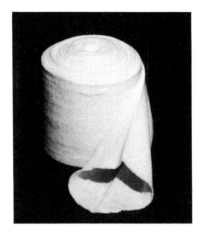

Figure 21

Plain cotton webbing is also used as a back cloth in the preparation of an elastic adhesive bandage. This is extremely useful where it is desired to maintain an even exertion of pressure over a relatively long period. The adhesive quality of the bandage prevents any slipping; once applied, it stays in place. This is known commercially as Ace Adhesive Bandage®. A new type of compression bandage incorporating the advantages of the Ace Adhesive Bandage®, but not sticking to the skin, is Peg®. This bandage sticks to itself and does not slip or loosen. An added advantage is that once applied, water does not loosen it, making it extremely useful in athletics.

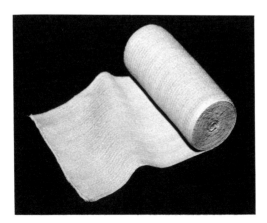

Figure 22

UNIT TWO ...

ELEMENTARY BANDAGING

CONTENTS OF UNIT TWO

Elementary Bandaging

Chapter 5
The Basic Turns

Chapter 6
Bandaging of Cylinders

Chapter 7
Bandaging of Cones

Chapter 8
Bandaging of Ovoids

Chapter 9
The Figure-of-Eight Turns

Chapter 10
Starting and Terminating of Bandages

Chapter 11
Axioms of Good Functional Bandaging

5

The Basic Turns

Definition

A basic turn may be defined as the unit of structure in a bandage. It represents a single encirclement of a part by the roller bandage, with return to the starting point, or to a point on a line with same. The direction taken by the roller in encircling the part serves as a basis of classification of the basic turns. All turns are begun by applying the external surface of the roller to the part to be bandaged.

Classification

There are only five basic turns, one, or more than one of which in combination, may be used to prepare any type of bandage on the body. These are:

1. Circular turns.
2. Spiral turns.
3. Spiral reverse turns.
4. Recurrent turns.
5. Figure-of-eight turns.

A better understanding of the mechanism of preparing these various turns will be obtained by demonstrating their adaptation to the basic figures of the body. It would be a relatively simple task merely to memorize which of the five basic turns is adaptable to each of the three simple figures; however, an attempt will be made, with the aid of a series of simple diagrams, to demonstrate why certain turns are adaptable to each of the basic figures. The functional bandager learns by under-standing and comprehension rather than by mere memory. Whereas one

27

often forgets that which he has memorized without comprehension, he is much less likely to forget that which he has learned by careful and logical explanation and understanding.

The succeeding chapters will be concerned with the bandaging of the *cylinder,* the *cone,* and the *ovoid.* The bandager would at all times do well to have available the "geometric configuration of the human body," so that as he learns the bandaging of the basic figures, he also begins to think in terms of the parts of the body represented by these basic figures. The transition from one to another then becomes a simple matter.

The *figure-of-eight turn,* although not necessary for bandaging any of the basic figures *per se,* is extremely valuable in bandaging points of junction of these figures, such as occur at the wrist, elbow, shoulder, hip, knee, and ankle. Thus, a separate chapter is devoted to the application of this turn. (See *The Figure-of-Eight Turns,* Chapter 9.)

6

Bandaging of Cylinders

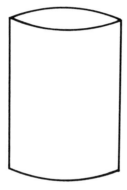

Figure 23

There are two main turns used in bandaging the cylinders of the body: (a) Circular turns, and (b) spiral turns.

CIRCULAR TURNS

In this type, having encircled the part, the roll of bandage returns to the exact point of starting, the second turn completely overlapping the first. The third turn completely overlaps the second. Thus, the area covered by the bandage is equal in width to the width of the roll of bandage.

Directions

(Note: These directions are for a right-handed person. If left-handed, use the hands opposite to those described in the following directions)

29

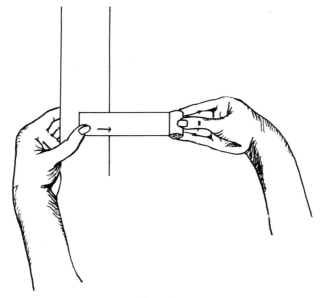

Figure 24

A. Hold the roller bandage in the right hand.

B. Lay the free edge of the bandage against the body surface to be bandaged, holding it in place with the left thumb. (See Fig. 24.) The external surface of the roller is applied to the part.

C. Carry the roller to the right with the right hand, making a clockwise turn.

D. Posteriorly transfer the roller to the left hand; with the right hand hold the beginning of the turn in place. (See Fig. 25.)

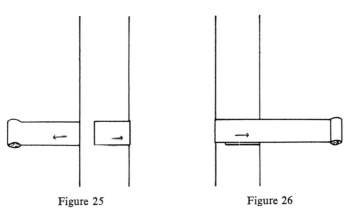

Figure 25   Figure 26

E. Carry the roller forward with the left hand, exactly covering the initial turn of the bandage. (See Fig. 26.)

This completes the first circular turn. The second circular turn is an exact duplication of the first.

Applications

The circular turn is best adapted for application to cylinder-shaped parts, such as the neck, the trunk, the wrists, and the lower leg. Since several circular turns fix a bandage securely, this basic turn is often used to anchor the material in the application of numerous types of bandages.

SPIRAL TURNS

It is obvious from the foregoing that the circular turn covers an area equal only to the width of the roll of bandage. To cover an area wider than the roll of bandage, spiral turns are used. In this type, each turn, instead of completely overlapping the previous turn as in the circular bandage, only partly overlaps the previous turn. The degree of overlapping varies from ½ to ⅔ to ¾ of the width of the bandage. By this method a bandage can be used to cover a surface much wider than the width of the material used.

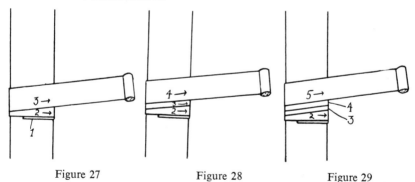

| Figure 27 | Figure 28 | Figure 29 |

Directions

A. Anchor the roller with one or two circular turns as described previously. (See Fig. 26.)

B. Begin the spiral as follows: Carry the bandage around again, but instead of completely overlapping the previous turn, carry it upward slightly; thus, when it returns to a point on a line with the starting point, it has progressed upward on the part. (See Fig. 27.)

The following turn, and each successive one, incompletely overlaps the previous one, and thus the bandage progresses upward to cover the entire part. (See Figs. 28, 29.)

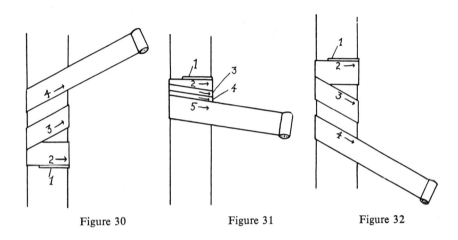

Figure 30   Figure 31   Figure 32

Classification of Spiral Turns

One can readily see from the foregoing explanations and illustrations that spiral turns which overlap the previous ones by ½ to ¾ the width of the material will naturally be slower in covering a part, and will require more material than will those which cover the previous turns by only ⅓ or ¼ of the width of the material. In fact, spiral turns may be so applied that the turns do not even overlap at all. These latter turns are referred to as *Rapid Ascending Spiral Turns,* in contrast to the previously described ones which are referred to as *Slow Ascending Spiral Turns.* (See Figs. 29, 30.)

Spiral turns may begin at an anatomically high point and then descend on an extremity, each turn overlapping the previous one as in the *Slow Ascending Spiral Turns.* These are then known as *Slow Descending Spiral Turns.* Similarly, the *Rapid Descending Spiral Turns* may be produced. (See Figs. 31, 32.)

Applications

The spiral turns are of value in covering a cylinder over an area which is greater in width than the width of the bandage material itself. These turns may also be utilized in bandaging cone-shaped parts which do not have too great a degree of angulation. Thus, the spiral is applicable to the lower parts of the forearm, arm, leg, thigh, fingers, toes, thorax, and abdomen. The limitations of the spiral in bandaging the cone will be discussed in the next chapter, *Bandaging of Cones.*

7

Bandaging of Cones

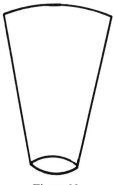

Figure 33

The cone presents a new problem, not encountered in bandaging the cylinder. Since the diameter of the cone gradually increases, if circular or even spiral turns were applied to the cone, the results would be as illustrated. (See Figs. 34, 35.) It will be noted in each of these illustrations that, although the upper border of the roller is firmly applied, the lower border is loose. This gives a "skirtlike" or "whiskerslike" effect to the lower border, and thus the bandage would rapidly fall off at the slightest tension, or contact with another surface. Thus, neither circular nor spiral turns can be used alone to good advantage on cones.

The turns best adapted for bandaging the cone are the Spiral Reverse Turns.

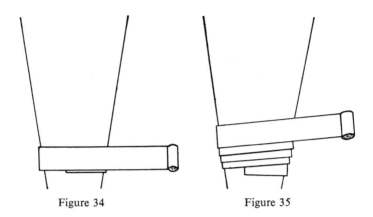

Figure 34   Figure 35

SPIRAL REVERSE TURNS

This turn derives its name as follows:

1. *Spiral:* The bandage proceeds upward on the cone in a spiral fashion, each turn only partly overlapping the preceding one.

2. *Reverse:* Instead of allowing the external surface of the bandage to be in contact with the cone throughout the bandage, as in the circular and spiral turns, the roller is reversed so that the internal surface comes into contact with the cone. In the next turn, there is a reverse again, and the external surface once again comes into contact with the cone. This alternating continues throughout the spiral reverse.

This type of turn is devised for taking up and preventing the slack on the lower border of the roller in bandaging cone-shaped parts.

Directions

A. Anchor the bandage with one or two circular turns, which serve to partly fix the bandage. (See Fig. 36.)

B. Proceed with the next turn as though beginning a spiral turn; that is, partly overlapping the previous one. The bandage should be applied at such an angle that no slack or "skirt" is allowed to develop at the lower border. Hold this turn in place with the left thumb. The thumb should be applied midway between the upper and lower borders of the bandage. (See Fig. 37.)

C. In the present position, the palm of the right hand (holding the roller) is facing upward (supinated). Unroll the bandage slightly to allow slack to develop between the point held by the left thumb and the roller. (See Fig. 37.)

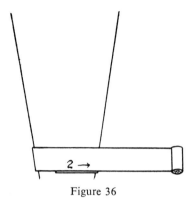

Figure 36

D. Turn the right palm downward (pronated) and, using the left thumb as a guide to hold the bandage in place, pass the bandage around the cone to complete the turn. (See Fig. 38.) This brings the inner surface into contact with the bandaged surface.

E. The next turn is a repetition of the first: (a) Begin spiral, partly overlapping the previous turn (See Fig. 39); (b) apply the left thumb to hold the bandage in place; (c) unroll the bandage to develop slack; (d) change the right hand from a position of supination to one of pronation and complete the turn (See Fig. 40); (e) repeat these turns until the part is covered (See Fig. 41.).

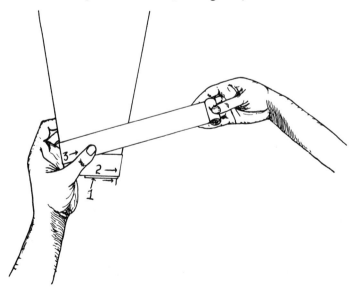

Figure 37

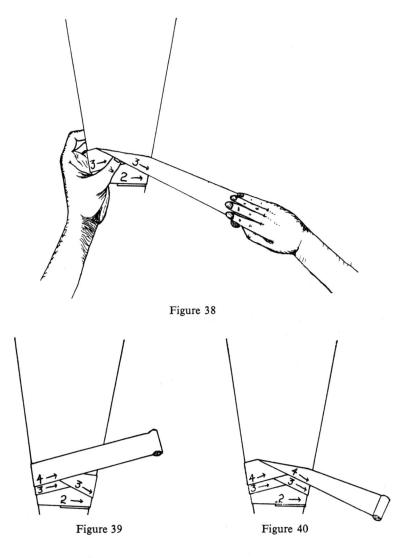

Figure 38

Figure 39   Figure 40

Although a properly executed spiral reverse turn is probably the most difficult maneuver in bandaging, there will be little difficulty in preparing perfect turns if the following points are adhered to:

1. The thumb should be placed midway between the upper and lower borders in each turn.

2. There should be plenty of slack between the body of the roller and the thumb holding the bandage in place as the reverse is executed.

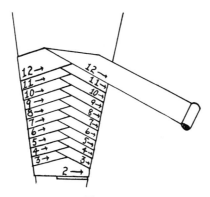

Figure 41

3. The material should fit snugly over the tip of the thumb as the reverse is completed.

4. The position of the thumb determines the point of crossing of the turns; thus, in each turn, the thumb should be applied directly above its position in the preceding turn; thus, a single straight line would pass through all points of crossing, making for a symmetrical bandage.

5. The attention should be focused, as the reverse is being completed and the slack taken up, upon maintaining a fixed and even distance between the borders of adjacent turns of bandage. Thus, if one examines the completed spiral reverse, it will be noted that both left and right sides of each turn are equal in width, thereby producing a symmetrical bandage.

Classification of Spiral Reverse Turns

The foregoing described spiral reverse is the "Ascending Spiral Reverse." Similarly, there is a "Descending Spiral Reverse" turn. The principles are exactly the same with the following modifications in the procedure:

1. After the initial fixing circular turn, the right hand receives the bandage with the palm downward (pronated). It will be remembered that in the Ascending Spiral Reverse the hand received the bandage with the palm upward.

2. The thumb holds the bandage in place, slack is allowed to develop, and the right hand is turned to make the palm face upward (supinated).

3. The turn is then completed.

Applications

    The spiral reverse turn is especially adaptable to those parts of the body which have gradually increasing or decreasing diameters. Thus, it is of value in the upper forearm, upper arm, upper leg, and thigh. Of course, the adaptation to various parts and the choice of the spiral reverse over the simple spiral will depend entirely upon the individual structure of the part. In a thin, poorly developed individual, the simple spiral would probably serve for bandaging an entire forearm; however, in a well developed, muscular individual, there is a marked increase in diameter from the lower to the upper forearm and thus the spiral reverse is necessary.

    Having mastered both spiral and spiral reverse turns, the bandager finds no difficulty in changing from one to the other as the necessity arises. After repeated practice, one sees at a glance at which point the change should be made. This makes for a smoothly executed and snug-fitting bandage.

8

Bandaging of Ovoids

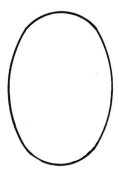

Figure 42

The main problems involved in bandaging the ovoid or rounded surfaces are twofold: (a) Adequate covering of the part, and (b) proper fixation of the bandage.

The circular, spiral, or spiral reverse turns, either alone or in combination, would not completely satisfy these requirements for bandaging a rounded surface.

The turns best adapted for bandaging the ovoid or rounded surfaces are the circular and recurrent turns, employed together. The circular turn has been previously described. (See Chapter 6.)

RECURRENT TURNS

In the recurrent turns, the bandage is passed over the tip of the ovoid. It is fixed at one point on the opposite side of the figure. It is then reflected upon itself so that it either exactly retraces its original course, or so that it diverges slightly from the point at which it is fixed. It is then brought back to the starting point, thus completing the first recurrent turn.

The following directions and illustrations will clarify and facilitate the performance of this turn.

Directions

A. Fix the bandage in place with one or two circular turns around the widest part of the ovoid. (See Figs. 43, 44.)

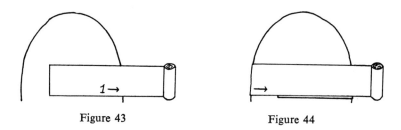

Figure 43   Figure 44

B. Fix the bandage at the center of the circular turn and pass the bandage over the center of the tip of the ovoid. Continue downward until the circular turn is reached on the opposite side of the ovoid. (See Figs. 45, 46.)

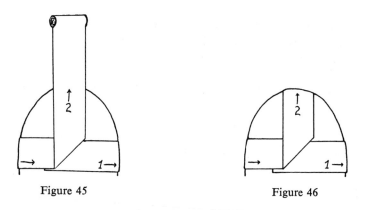

Figure 45   Figure 46

C. Fix the bandage in place on the opposite side, and bring the bandage back to the original point, only partly overlapping the first turn. This completes the first recurrent turn. (See Fig. 47.)

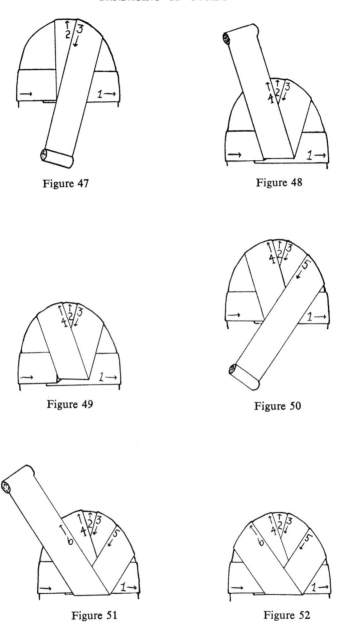

Figure 47

Figure 48

Figure 49

Figure 50

Figure 51

Figure 52

D. The next recurrent turn is exactly similar to the first, except that in each successive turn, the bandage only partly overlaps the previous one. In doing the recurrents, if one turn passes to the left of the midline, the next should pass to the right of the midline, and thus the

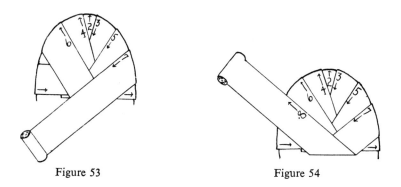

Figure 53   Figure 54

turns alternate. In this manner, the turns diverge from the center of the ovoid, eventually covering the entire surface. (See Figs. 48, 49, 50, 51, 52, 53, 54.)

E. When the entire surface has been covered, fix the ends in place by a few circular turns. (See Fig. 55.)

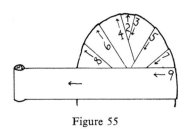

Figure 55

In applying the recurrent turns, it is advisable to have either the patient or an assistant hold the ends in place until the final circular turns have been applied.

Applications

The main ovoids in the body to which the recurrent turn is applicable are: (a) The head, (b) tips of fingers, (c) tips of toes, (d) amputation stumps, and (e) the hand when closed to form a fist. Although the latter four are only partial ovoids, the principles are essentially the same.

9

The Figure-of-Eight Turns

Introduction

Although the four basic turns previously described may be used to cover the three fundamental geometric figures comprising the human body, there often arises the necessity for the application of the fifth basic turn, the figure-of-eight. In fact, the figure-of-eight turn is probably used as frequently as any other turn since it is more subject to variations and adapts itself more readily to a number of different purposes and circumstances. By some it is regarded as the most valuable of the fundamental turns.

As the name implies, these turns take the form of the figure *eight,* consisting of two loops and one point of crossing; thus, a dressing may be held in place, or special compression made, by either of the loops or by the point of crossing.

Directions

The following illustrations show the preparation of a single figure-of-eight turn. From the initial extremity the bandage proceeds upward and encircles the part. It is then brought downward to cross the initial extremity at an oblique angle. It is then continued around the part, and then returned to the starting point. (See Figs. 56, 57, 58, 59, 60.)

Classification of Figure-of-Eight Turns

The figure-of-eight turn illustrated is the simple basic turn. The next figure-of-eight turn may vary in its relation to the first, and this variation in the relative position of subsequent turns serves as a basis of classification of the figure-of-eight turns, thus:

43

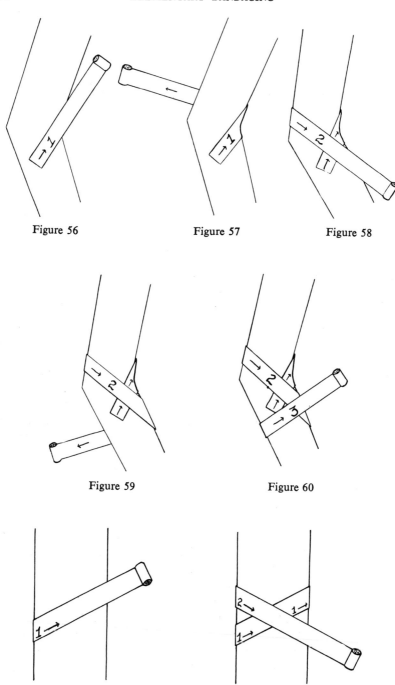

Figure 56   Figure 57   Figure 58

Figure 59   Figure 60

Figure 61   Figure 62

1. The turns may ascend, to form Ascending Figure-of-eights. The turns proceed upwards on the part, each turn only partly overlapping and lying higher than the previous one. (See Figs. 61, 62, 63, 64, 65, 66.)

2. The turns may descend, to form the Descending Figure-of-eight. The turns proceed downward, each turn only partly overlapping and lying lower than the previous one. (See Figs. 67, 68, 69, 70, 71, 72.)

3. The turns may diverge from a central point to form the Divergent or Eccentric Figure-of-eight. (See Figs. 73, 74, 75, 76, 77, 78.)

4. The turns may converge toward a central point to form the Concentric Figure-of-eight.

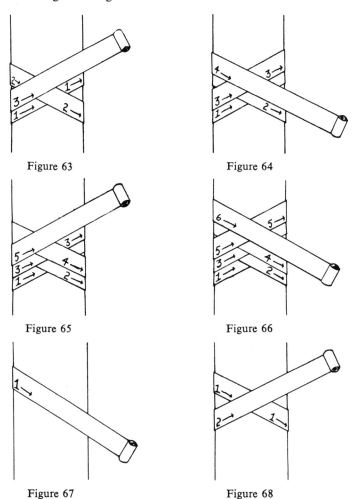

Figure 63   Figure 64

Figure 65   Figure 66

Figure 67   Figure 68

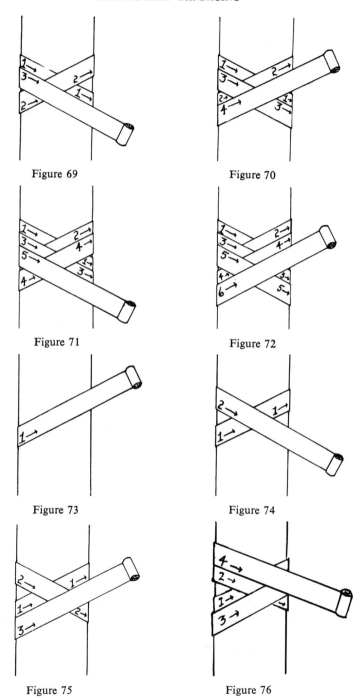

Figure 69

Figure 70

Figure 71

Figure 72

Figure 73

Figure 74

Figure 75

Figure 76

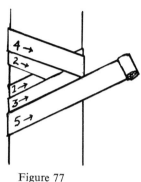

Figure 77

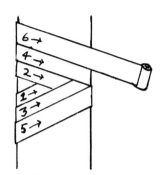

Figure 78

INDICATIONS FOR THE USE OF THE FIGURE-OF-EIGHT TURNS

The figure-of-eight is used in bandaging regions of the body to which the previously described turns are not readily adaptable. The figure-of-eight is used for bandaging:

1. *Joints:* The elbow, the knee, the wrist, and the ankle.

2. *Junctions of the Extremities with the Trunk:* The shoulder (arm and thorax), the hip (thigh and lower abdomen).

3. *Special Junctions of a Narrow and a Wider Part:* Thumb and the wrist, head and neck.

4. *Cone-shaped Parts:* As a substitute for the spiral reverse turns.

THE SPICA BANDAGES

Figure-of-eight bandages in which one loop is of greater circumference than the other and in which the points of crossing of succeeding turns form sharp or steep angles are called *spica bandages.* This is derived from the resemblance of these bandages to the husks of an ear of corn. (See Fig. 8, *Spica of Groin.*)

REGIONAL BANDAGING WITH THE FIGURE-OF-EIGHT

Further application of the figure-of-eight will be demonstrated in the special section on *Regional Bandaging.*

10

Starting and Terminating of Bandages

Starting of Bandages

Proper fixation of the initial extremity of the roller is of utmost importance in the application of all bandages. Unless this extremity is adequately anchored, it will be found that when tension is applied to subsequent turns, the bandage begins to slip, instead of remaining firmly applied to the part.

The most commonly used method for initial fixation of a bandage is the application of several circular turns to a cylinder-shaped part. (See Fig. 79.) Additional methods include:

1. OBLIQUE FIXATION

In this method, the initial extremity is crossed obliquely by the first turn. (See Fig. 80.) This method is often used in the starting of figure-of-eight bandages.

2. ADHESIVE PLASTER FIXATION

A strip of adhesive plaster, about three inches long and one inch wide, is applied partly upon the bandage and partly upon the skin. This fixes the bandage. (See Fig. 81.) This is then covered with one circular turn of the bandage.

CONTINUATION OF A BANDAGE WITH A SECOND ROLLER

Occasionally, a roller of bandage is too short for a particular dressing. The initial extremity of the second roller is applied directly over the terminal extremity of the first, and one to two circular turns are then applied. This fixes the second roller, and the bandage is then continued.

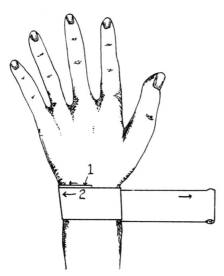

Figure 79

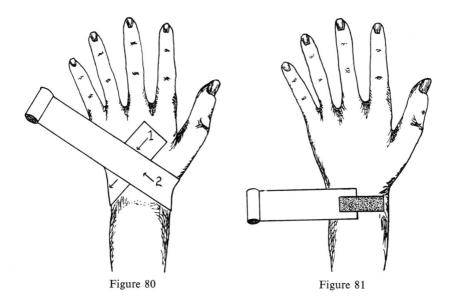

Figure 80   Figure 81

Terminating of Bandages
INTRODUCTION

A well executed bandage must have secure fixation of its terminal extremity; otherwise, the entire bandage is rendered useless. A loosely fixed terminal extremity may lead to loosening of the entire bandage, thereby resulting in loss of time, effort, and effectiveness. A variety of methods may be used, the choice to depend on the availability of material and the discretion of the bandager.

The methods employed, in the order of frequency of application, are:

1. Tying with the roller itself.
2. Fixing with adhesive plaster.
3. Pinning with safety pins.
4. Tucking end of bandage underneath
   the previous turn; and
5. Sewing.

1. Tying with the Roller, Itself: There are several methods for using the gauze roller to fix the bandage in place.

A. *Splitting of Terminal Extremity:* The terminal extremity of the bandage is split. (See Figs. 82, 83.) The ends are then passed around the part in opposite directions and tied. It is important in this method, in order to prevent the bandage from tearing further and becoming loose, to pass the ends in a proper manner. That end which is to travel in a direction opposite to the direction of the bandage (End *B*—See Fig. 84) is first passed underneath the other end (End *A*—See Fig. 84), which is to continue in the direction of the bandage. The ends are then carried in their respective directions and tied. (See Fig. 85.)

A modification of this method is the following: After the end of the bandage has been split, the two newly formed ends (*A* and *B*) are tied with a single knot. This prevents further splitting of the material. The two ends are then carried around the part in opposite directions and tied.

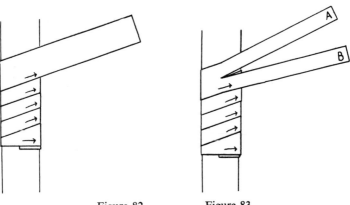

Figure 82   Figure 83

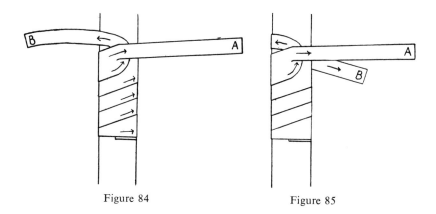

Figure 84   Figure 85

B. *Full Width Tie* (Bellevue Tie): At the completion of the
last turn, the roller is in the right hand. The bandage is unwound for
a short distance and some slack is allowed to develop. The left hand
grasps the portion where the slack has developed (See Fig. 86) and the
right hand then carries the roller in a counterclockwise fashion, opposite to its direction on the last turn. (See Fig. 87.) This makes for a
double fold of material in the left hand. When the right hand completes its
counterclockwise turn, there is presented a single fold in the right hand
which can then be tied to the double fold in the left hand. (See Fig. 88.)

2. Fixing with Adhesive Plaster Strips: At the completion of the last
turn of a bandage, the material is cut from the roller. A strip of adhesive
plaster, about three inches long and one inch wide, is applied with half
on the last turn and half on the previous turn. (See Fig. 89.)

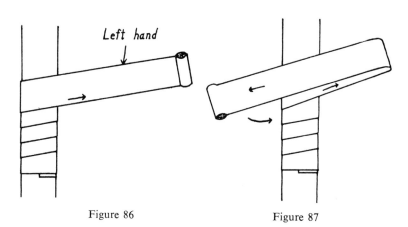

Figure 86   Figure 87

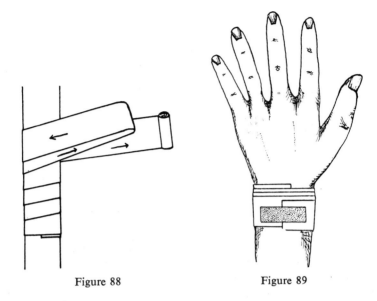

Figure 88   Figure 89

3. Pinning with Safety Pins: The last turn of a bandage may be fixed by pinning it to the underlying previous turn. Pins may be applied in either of two ways:

A. *Crosswise:* In this method, the long axis of the pin is at right angles to the direction of the bandage. (See Fig. 90.) The advantage of this method is that the pull is divided into two axes of direction, and thus there is less strain upon the threads.

B. *Lengthwise:* In this method, the long axis of the pin is in the same axis as the direction of the bandage. (See Fig. 91.) The disadvantage of this method is that the pull is along one axis, and the threads of material along this axis are under a greater strain than in the previously described method, in which the tension is divided.

4. Folding the Last Turn Under the Previous One: At the completion of the last turn, the material is pulled slightly tighter than usual, and the end is tucked under the upper border of the previous turn. This method has the disadvantage that if there is too much manipulation, or movement of the part, the bandage may come loose.

5. Sewing: When it is desired to maintain a dressing in place for some time, the last turn may be sewed to the underlying one by a few stitches through the terminal extremity. This method of fixation is rarely used.

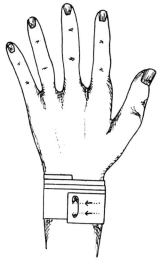

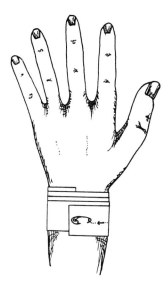

Figure 90   Figure 91

11

Axioms of Good Functional Bandaging

It is usually the very obvious which is so readily overlooked and thus the bandager often commits errors for which there is no justification. Were he to bear in mind certain very simple basic facts related to the subject of bandaging, there would be little cause for lament over errors. A list of truisms or axioms of bandaging is herein included, a knowledge of which will at all times serve the bandager in good stead. The alert and observing bandager will have many more to add as a result of repeated experience and observation.

1. "That sort of bandaging is the worst which quickly falls off; but those are bad bandages which neither compress nor yet come off." (Hippocrates)

2. When wet, bandages shrink and become tighter, constricting the part and interfering with the circulation.

3. When the swelling goes down, the bandage becomes loose.

4. A poorly applied bandage is uneconomical, since it requires too frequent change.

5. Any bandage which leaves a considerable portion of the distal extremity of a limb uncovered is liable to induce swelling. Once started, it progresses rapidly since it increases the tension of the lower border of the bandage.

6. In applying bandages to the chest, care must be observed that respiration is not interfered with, particularly if the dressing is completed before the patient has recovered from the effects of an anesthetic.

7. Bandages should not be applied directly to a wound.

8. The surface of the bandage should lie flat on the bandaged part.

9. In bandaging an extremity, it is advisable, if possible, to leave a small portion of the extremity exposed, so that any change in circulation may be detected.

10. Skin surfaces should not be in contact in a bandage. Thus, when two fingers are bandaged together, or an arm is bandaged in front of the chest, all points where two surfaces meet should be protected by some material, such as gauze or lint or cotton wadding.

UNIT THREE ...

ADVANCED REGIONAL BANDAGING

*"The growth of knowledge may be likened
to the ascent of a spiral stair from which the
observer periodically surveys the same landscape,
but each time from a higher level than the last."*

Sir Michael Foster

CONTENTS OF UNIT THREE

Advanced Regional Bandaging

Chapter 12

Introduction to Advanced Regional Bandaging

Chapter 13

Bandages for the Upper Extremity

Chapter 14

Bandages for the Lower Extremity

Chapter 15

Bandages for the Head, Face, and Neck

Chapter 16

Bandages for the Neck, Chest, and Axilla

Chapter 17

Bandages for the Chest and Abdomen

Chapter 18

Bandages for the Breasts

Chapter 19

Bandages for the Arm, Chest, and Shoulder

Chapter 20

Bandages for the Groin, Perineum, and Buttock

12

Introduction to Advanced Regional Bandaging

To this point we have dealt with the basic turns of bandaging as applied to the three fundamental figures of which the body is constructed. The ease of transition from the cylinder, the cone, and the ovoid to corresponding parts of the human body now becomes apparent. (See Figs. 92, 93.)

In the approach to the bandaging of any region, one should first quickly visualize the part in terms of its geometric configuration; i.e., the wrist as a *cylinder,* the forearm as a *cone,* the head as an *ovoid,* etc. The basic turns to be applied to each of these figures have become "automatic" as it were. Then, with the fundamental principles of anatomy and physiology in mind, one proceeds to bandage the part.

In the application of bandages to living tissues, there are certain points of importance which cannot be too strongly emphasized.

The bandage must not be too tight, or too loose. A loose bandage neither stays in place, nor does it serve its purpose. A tight bandage constricts the part and interferes with the circulation, and thereby, the healing.

The methods of the bandager should be flexible, rather than rigid. Thus, a part which in a muscular individual requires a spiral reverse, may be bandaged, in the leaner individual, by simple spiral turns. The bandager should individualize his work.

The type of turn used should depend upon and vary, whenever possible, with the purpose for which it is applied: Thus, to apply a slow ascending spiral turn to hold a wet dressing in place is a waste of

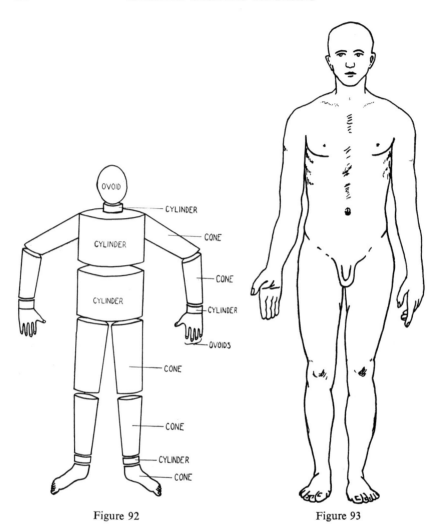

Figure 92   Figure 93

material if a rapid ascending spiral could serve the same purpose. A minimum of bandaging material should be used, making for greater economy.

All bandages should be well anchored by several circular turns, preferably over a cylinder-shaped part. Other previously described methods of anchoring bandages may be used as well.

The type of material should be of the proper texture and strength for both the part bandaged and for the purpose and function of the bandage. The patient certainly will be grateful for the application of softer materials to more sensitive and delicate parts.

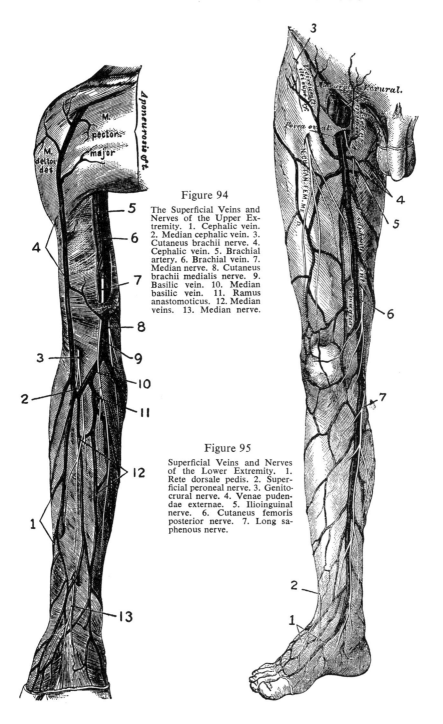

Figure 94

The Superficial Veins and Nerves of the Upper Extremity. 1. Cephalic vein. 2. Median cephalic vein. 3. Cutaneus brachii nerve. 4. Cephalic vein. 5. Brachial artery. 6. Brachial vein. 7. Median nerve. 8. Cutaneus brachii medialis nerve. 9. Basilic vein. 10. Median basilic vein. 11. Ramus anastomoticus. 12. Median veins. 13. Median nerve.

Figure 95

Superficial Veins and Nerves of the Lower Extremity. 1. Rete dorsale pedis. 2. Superficial peroneal nerve. 3. Genito-crural nerve. 4. Venae pudendae externae. 5. Ilioinguinal nerve. 6. Cutaneus femoris posterior nerve. 7. Long saphenous nerve.

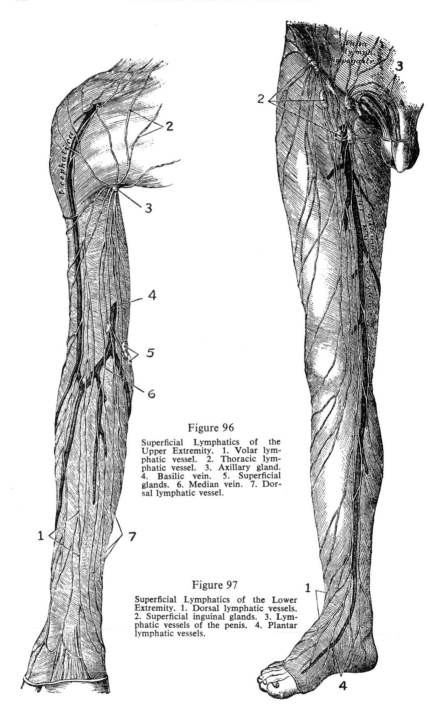

Figure 96

Superficial Lymphatics of the
Upper Extremity. 1. Volar lymphatic vessel. 2. Thoracic lymphatic vessel. 3. Axillary gland.
4. Basilic vein. 5. Superficial
glands. 6. Median vein. 7. Dorsal lymphatic vessel.

Figure 97

Superficial Lymphatics of the Lower
Extremity. 1. Dorsal lymphatic vessels.
2. Superficial inguinal glands. 3. Lymphatic vessels of the penis. 4. Plantar
lymphatic vessels.

Anatomico-physiological Application of Bandages

Bandaging and the application of various surgical dressings must be physiological as well as anatomical. The mere covering of a part of the body by a dressing, or bandage may be considered *anatomical*. This, alone, is not sufficient. There must be recognition of, and regard for, the structure and functions of the deeper-lying tissues. This is *physiological*.

Directly beneath the skin, and in the deeper layers as well, there is a thick bed of venous and lymphatic channels conveying blood and lymph from the periphery to the more proximal parts. (See Figs. 94, 95, 96, 97.)

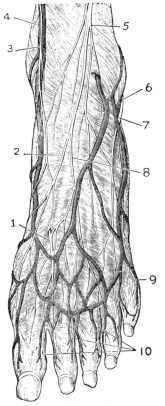

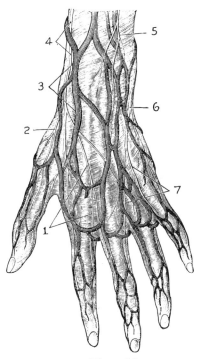

Figure 98

The Nerves at the Dorsum of the Foot.
1. Superficial peroneal nerve. 2. Cutaneus dorsalic intermedius nerve. 3. Internal saphenous nerve. 4. Internal saphenous vein. 5. Superficial peroneal nerve. 6. External saphenous vein. 7. Sural nerve. 8. Cutaneus dorsalis medialis nerve. 9. External dorsalis nerve. 10. Dorsal nerves.

Figure 99

The Nerves at the Dorsal Side of the Hand. 1. Dorsal nerves and radial nerve. 2. Dorsal nerves. 3. Cephalic vein. 4. Superfiicial radial nerve. 5. Cutaneus antibrachii medialis nerve. 6. Ulnar nerve. 7. Dorsal nerves and ulnar nerve.

It can readily be understood how a tightly applied bandage may constrict these channels and interfere with the return flow. This would lead to congestion and swelling. The greater the swelling at the distal border of a bandage, the greater the degree of constriction. Thus more channels become obstructed and so a vicious cycle is set up. This process may finally lead to interference with the arterial blood flow to the part, with resultant dire effects. Pressure on the peripheral nerves, so profusely distributed to the skin, leads to considerable pain. (See Figs. 98, 99.)

The skeletal and muscular structure of a part must be considered. Bony points, protected by only a thin layer of skin, as over the elbow, need special care and protection. The skin in these areas is exposed to much pressure and friction, and, unless given due care, may become irritated, inflamed, and ulcerated.

A bandage or surgical dressing is applied to living, nonstatic structures. For successful bandaging one must remember that blood and lymph flow, nerve impulses travel, muscles contract, and often bones move beneath the dressing. The dressing must encourage rather than interfere with the normal and reparative functions of these vital components.

13

Bandages for the Upper Extremity

1. Anatomico-physiological structure.
2. General principles.
3. Bandaging the wrist.
4. Bandaging the palm and dorsum of the hand.
5. Bandaging the fingers.
6. Bandaging the thumb.
7. Bandaging the forearm.
8. Bandaging the arm.
9. Bandaging the elbow.

1. ANATOMICO-PHYSIOLOGICAL STRUCTURE

The more superficial structures of the upper extremity, namely, the nerves, veins, and lymphatics, have been presented in the previous chapter. A pictorial summary is herein presented of the basic deeper structures: The muscles, whose individual patterns and degree of development are responsible for the particular contour of the parts, and the arteries, whose conveyance of blood with its nutritional elements is so necessary for both normal function and repair of injured tissues. (See Figs. 102, 103, 104.)

2. GENERAL PRINCIPLES

The wrist may be regarded as a starting point for most of the bandages of the upper extremity. Being cylindrical in shape, it is used for the application of anchoring circular turns. From this point one may

65

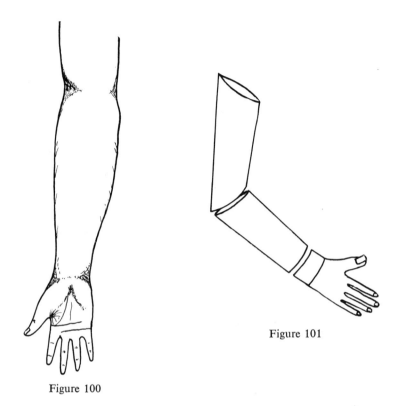

Figure 101

Figure 100

proceed to the fingers, the hand, the forearm, and higher. The importance of well anchored bandages in this region is well appreciated when one considers the degree of activity of the upper extremity as well as the contact with wearing apparel.

3. BANDAGING THE WRIST (two-inch bandage)

The wrist is a cylinder and is bandaged with simple circular turns. (See Fig. 105.) One or more spiral turns may be applied when it is desired to cover an area slightly wider than the width of the bandage used.

4. BANDAGING THE PALM AND THE DORSUM OF THE HAND (two-inch bandage)

The palm and the dorsum of the hand may be bandaged as a simple cylinder, with circular turns. However, in view of the tendency of such a bandage to slip off, it is advisable first to anchor the bandage at the

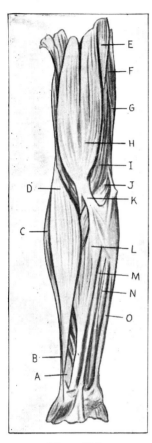

Figure 102

Muscles of Arm and Forearm, Anterior Aspect. A. Pronator quadratus. B. Abductor pollicis longus. C. Radial extensors. D. Brachioradialis. E. Coracobrachialis. F. Scapular head of triceps. G. Medial head of triceps. H. Biceps. I. Brachialis. J. Pronator teres, superior head. K. Bicipital aponeurosis. L. Flexor carpi radialis. M. Palmaris longus. N. Flexor digiti sublimis. O. Flexor carpi ulnaris.

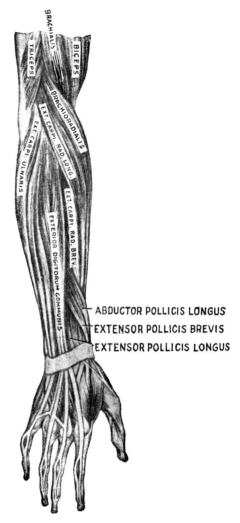

Figure 103

Extensor Muscles of Forearm.

wrist with a few circular turns, proceed to the palm, apply a few circular turns, and then return to the wrist. This method serves the purpose well; however, the ideal bandage for either the palm or the dorsum of the hand is the figure-of-eight bandage, with the points of crossing over the dorsum of the hand.

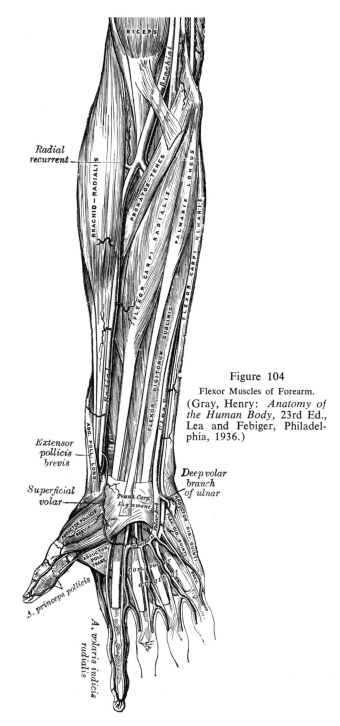

Figure 104

Flexor Muscles of Forearm.
(Gray, Henry: *Anatomy of the Human Body*, 23rd Ed., Lea and Febiger, Philadelphia, 1936.)

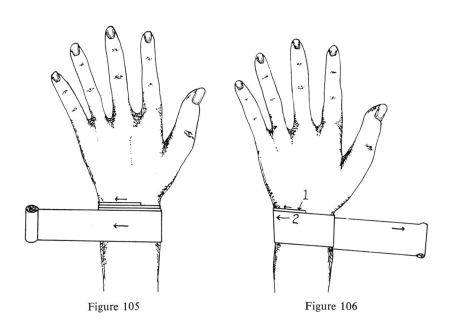

Figure 105   Figure 106

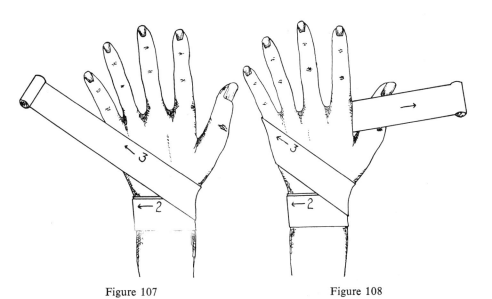

Figure 107   Figure 108

Directions

    A. Apply two circular turns around the wrist, terminating at the dorsum of the wrist. (See Fig. 106.)

    B. Carry the roller across the back of the hand (See Fig. 107), around the palm (See Fig. 108), back across the dorsum (See Fig. 109), and return to the wrist, completing the first figure-of-eight. (See Fig. 110.)

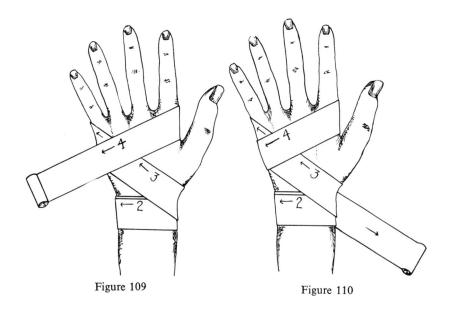

Figure 109   Figure 110

    C. Repeat with as many figure-of-eight turns as are necessary to cover adequately the dorsum or the palm. (See Fig. 111.)

    D. Terminate with one or two circular turns around the wrist. (See Fig. 112.)

THE DEMI-GAUNTLET BANDAGE (one-inch bandage)

    This is a bandage often used for dressing the dorsum of the hand, its main advantage being that the palm of the hand is not covered, allowing for free use of the palmar surface of the hand. The demi-gauntlet consists of a series of figure-of-eight turns around the wrist and bases of the fingers, with the points of crossing over the dorsum of the hand.

Directions

    A. Apply one or two circular turns around the wrist, completing the turns at the back of the wrist. (See Fig. 113.)

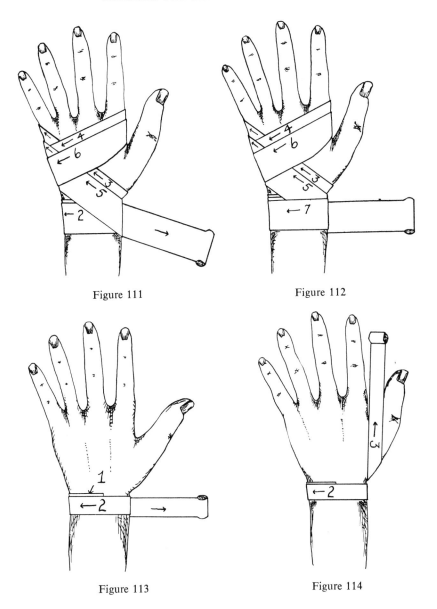

Figure 111

Figure 112

Figure 113

Figure 114

B. Carry the roller to the base of the nearest digit, the thumb, and encircle same, returning to the dorsum of the finger. (See Figs. 114, 115.)

C. Bring the roller back to the wrist and encircle it, thereby completing the first figure-of-eight. (See Fig. 116.)

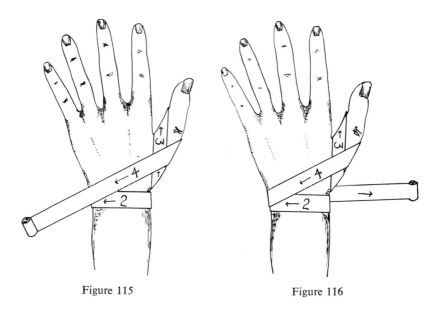

Figure 115　　　　　　　　　　　Figure 116

D. Carry the roller to the base of the next digit. (See Fig. 117.) Encircle the digit and return to the wrist, completing the second figure-of-eight. (See Figs. 118, 119.)

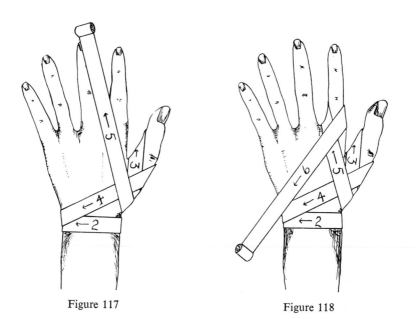

Figure 117　　　　　　　　　　　Figure 118

E. Proceed with the next three digits in a similar manner and terminate with one or two circular turns around the wrist. (See Fig. 120.)

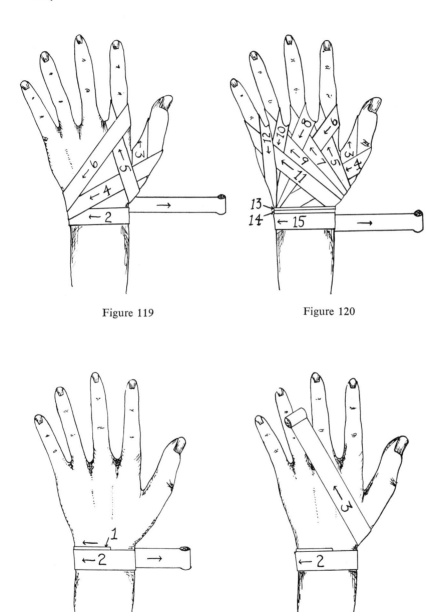

Figure 119

Figure 120

Figure 121

Figure 122

5. BANDAGING THE FINGERS (one-inch bandage)

The finger consists of two geometric figures. The tip of the finger is part of an ovoid, and requires recurrent turns. The body of the finger is usually a cylinder and is bandaged with spiral turns. Occasionally, however, the body of the finger assumes the shape of a gradually tapering cone, in this case requiring spiral reverse turns. The choice between spiral and spiral reverse turns will depend upon the judgment of the bandager.

A bandage for a finger is first anchored at the wrist, and then carried to the finger. The latter is bandaged and the bandage returned to, and fixed at, the wrist.

Directions

A. Anchor bandage with one or two circular turns around the wrist. (See Fig. 121.)

B. Carry roller across the dorsum of the hand to the base of the finger. (See Fig. 122.)

C. With a rapid descending spiral, carry roller to the end of the finger. (See Fig. 123.)

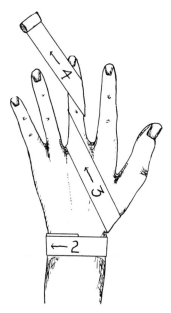

Figure 123

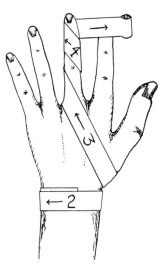

Figure 124

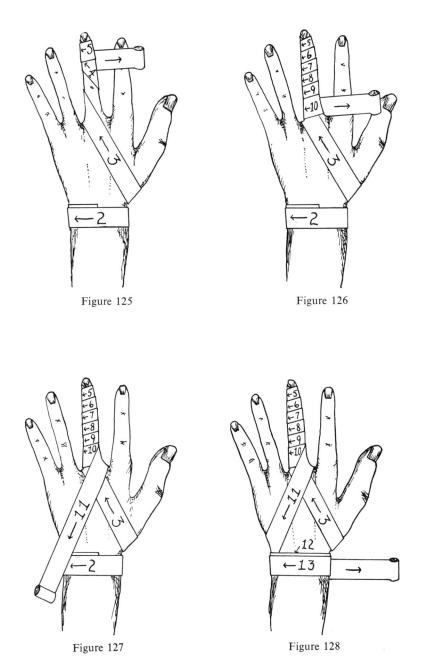

Figure 125

Figure 126

Figure 127

Figure 128

D. From this point, the bandage will vary, depending upon whether or not it is desired to cover the tip of the finger.

(a) If only the body of the finger is to be bandaged, then, having reached the end of the finger, carry the roller up the finger with slow ascending spiral turns, or, if these are not applicable, use spiral reverse turns. (See Figs. 124, 125, 126.) Having reached the base of the finger, carry the roller back over the dorsum of the hand to the wrist (See Fig. 127), and complete with one or two circular turns here. (See Fig. 128.)

(b) If the tip of the finger is to be covered, the procedure is similar to the above, except that recurrent turns are applied to the tip. The first recurrent turn is applied by merely continuing the descending spiral over the center of the nail. (See Figs. 129, 130.)

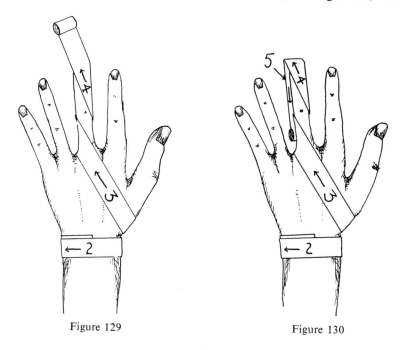

Figure 129   Figure 130

The second recurrent turn passes slightly to one side of the first (See Figs. 131, 132) and the third to the other side of the first. (See Figs. 133, 134.) This creates at the fingertip an arrow-shaped covering which makes it possible to cover easily the borders of the recurrent turns as the spirals are begun. (See Fig. 134.) The roller is brought to the fingertip again (See Fig. 135) and the slow ascending spiral is begun. (See Fig. 136.) These turns are continued to the base of the finger, and then the procedure is completed as above. (See Figs. 137, 138.)

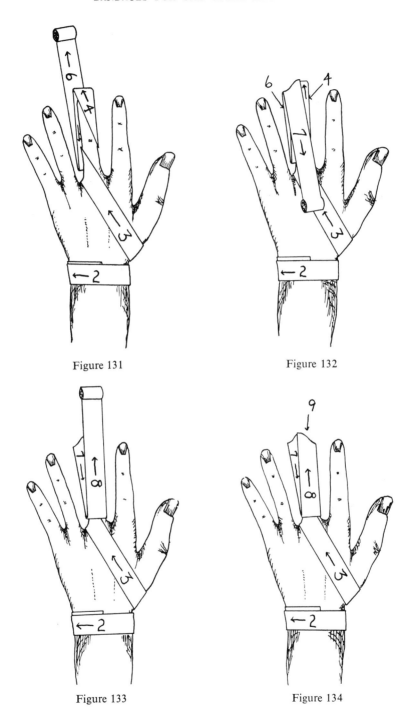

Figure 131

Figure 132

Figure 133

Figure 134

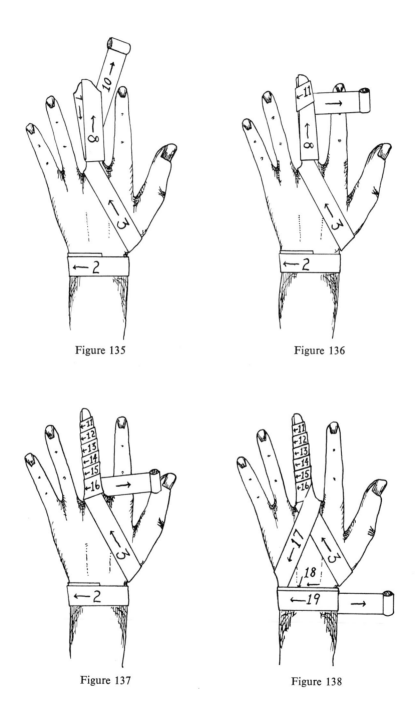

Figure 135   Figure 136

Figure 137   Figure 138

VARIATIONS IN FINGER BANDAGES

The foregoing described bandages may be applied to more than one finger of the same hand. Thus, after one finger is bandaged, and the wrist encircled with one or two circular turns, the roller is again brought across the dorsum of the hand to the base of the next finger. The latter is bandaged as was the first, and the roller returned to the wrist. (See Fig. 139.) Two or three fingers may be bandaged as one in a common bandage; however, it must be remembered that skin surfaces in contact must be protected with some intervening material.

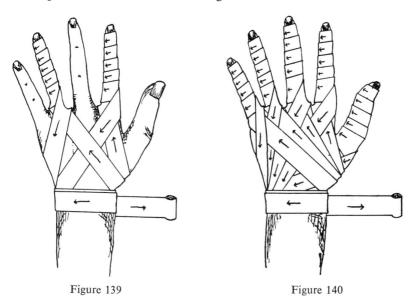

Figure 139   Figure 140

THE GAUNTLET BANDAGE (one-inch bandage)

The gauntlet bandage is merely a combination of the finger bandages and the semi-gauntlet. (See Fig. 120.) As the bandage reaches the base of each finger, instead of merely encircling the base of the finger and returning to the wrist, the entire finger is first bandaged, and then the roller is returned to the wrist. Thus all of the fingers are bandaged in rotation. (See Fig. 140.)

6. BANDAGING THE THUMB (one-inch bandage)

The thumb may be bandaged as any of the other fingers of the hand, as previously described. Anchored first at the wrist, the bandage is brought to the thumb. The latter is bandaged with spiral, or spiral reverse, turns and the bandage returned to the wrist where it is fixed.

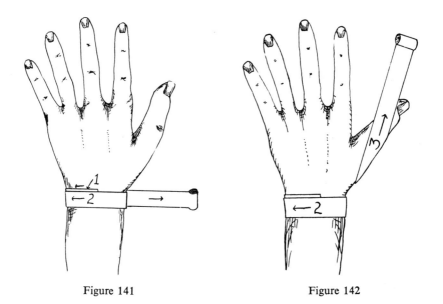

Figure 141   Figure 142

A much firmer and more effective type of bandage for the thumb is the ascending figure-of-eight, often referred to as the *Spica of the Thumb*. This consists of a series of figure-of-eight turns around the thumb and wrist.

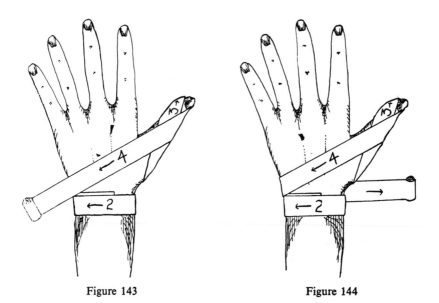

Figure 143   **Figure 144**

Directions

A. Anchor the bandage with one or two circular turns around the wrist. (See Fig. 141.)

B. Carry the roller across the dorsum of the thumb to the tip of the finger. (See Fig. 142.)

C. Encircle the tip of the thumb and carry the roller across the dorsum of the hand. (See Fig. 143.)

D. Encircle the wrist, thereby completing the first figure-of-eight. (See Fig. 144.)

E. Encircle the thumb again, only partly overlapping the first turn, and return to the wrist, completing the second figure-of-eight. (See Figs. 145, 146.)

F. Repeat with as many more figures-of-eight as are necessary to completely cover the thumb. (See Fig. 147.)

G. Terminate the bandage with one or two circular turns around the wrist. (See Fig. 148.)

7. BANDAGING THE FOREARM (two- and three-inch bandages)

The forearm is represented as a cone. The lower portion of the forearm, just above the wrist, however, closely approximates the cylinder in shape. Thus, having anchored the bandage at the wrist, one proceeds upward on the forearm using the simple spiral turns. When a point is reached at which the forearm widens fairly rapidly, that is, in the upper

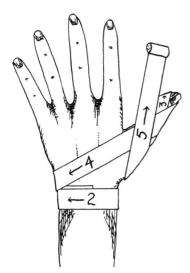

Figure 145

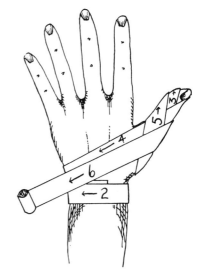

Figure 146

forearm, the spiral reverse is used. The point of transition from the spiral to the spiral reverse is quickly recognized by the alert bandager. Often, particularly in thin individuals, or those with poor muscular development, it is possible to bandage the entire forearm with merely a simple spiral bandage. This depends entirely upon the judgment of the bandager.

Directions

A. Anchor the bandage with one or two circular turns around the wrist. (See Fig. 149.)

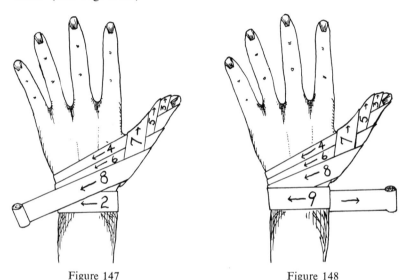

Figure 147   Figure 148

B. With slow ascending spiral turns, proceed upward on the arm. (See Fig. 150.)

C. At the point at which small "skirts" begin to appear at the lower border of the bandage, revert to the spiral reverse. (See Fig. 151.)

D. Continue the spiral reverse until the part is covered. (See Fig. 152.)

8. BANDAGING THE ARM (two- and three-inch bandages)

The arm is a cone and is bandaged with spiral reverse turns. Occasionally, when not developed, the arm may be bandaged with simple spiral turns.

Directions

A. Anchor the bandage with one or two circular turns just above the elbow. (See Fig. 153.)

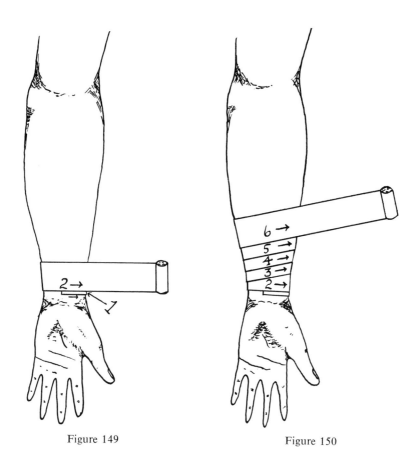

Figure 149   Figure 150

B. Proceed upward with either spiral or spiral reverse turns, depending upon the contour of the part, until the arm is covered. (See Figs. 154, 155.)

C. Complete with one or two circular turns. (See Fig. 156.)

9. BANDAGING THE ELBOW (three-inch bandage)

In bandaging the upper extremity in a position of extension, the elbow region is covered as are the arm and forearm, with either spiral, or spiral reverse turns, depending upon which of these is more adaptable. However, in bandaging the elbow in a position of flexion, the figure-of-eight, or spica bandage, is used. Since the point of the elbow is most difficult to cover, it is covered first, and then eccentric, or divergent, figure-of-eight turns are applied.

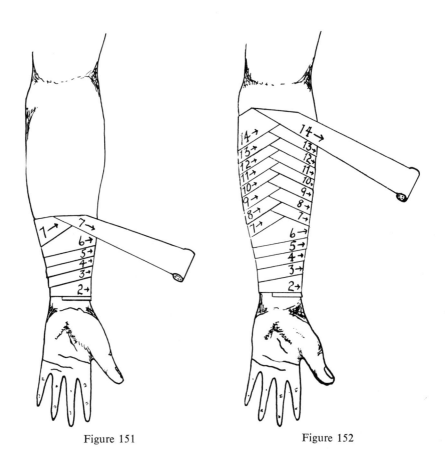

Figure 151   Figure 152

Directions

A. Apply one or two circular and spiral turns to the upper forearm to anchor the bandage. (See Fig. 157.)

B. Apply a circular turn around the point of the elbow. (See Fig. 158.)

C. Start the first figure-of-eight turn by a loop around the upper forearm. This turn should overlap the lower border of the circular turn around the point of the elbow. (See Fig. 159.)

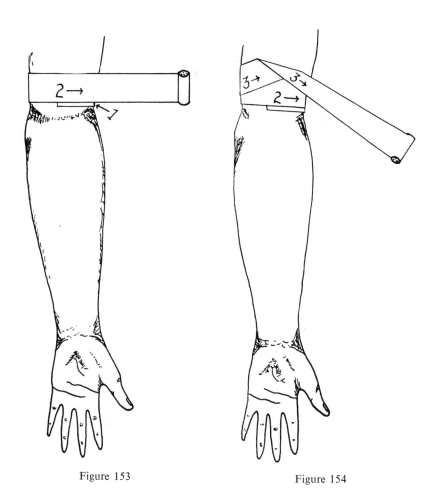

Figure 153   Figure 154

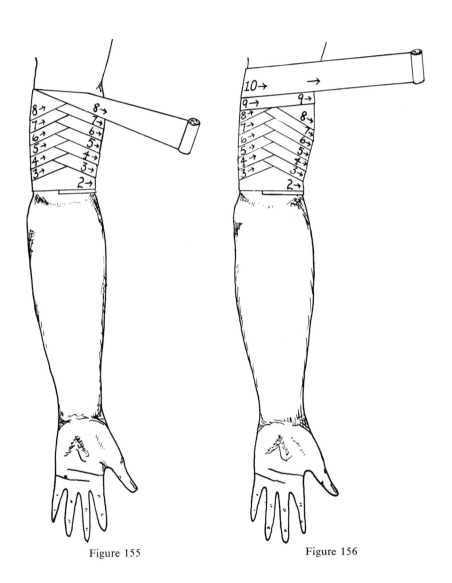

Figure 155   Figure 156

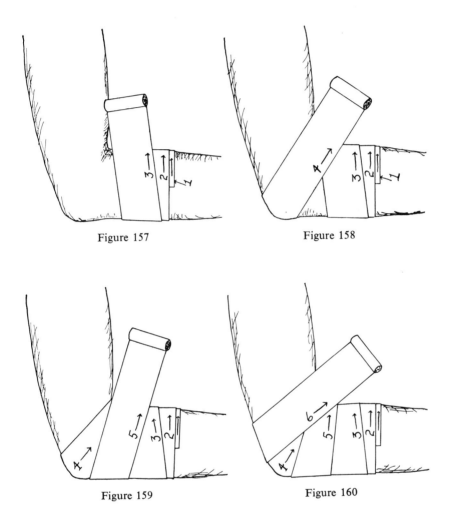

Figure 157   Figure 158

Figure 159   Figure 160

D. Apply the second loop of the figure-of-eight turn around the lower arm. This turn should overlap the upper border of the circular turn around the elbow. (See Fig. 160.) Thus, this first figure-of-eight turn serves to fix the circular turn which covers the point of the elbow.

E. Continue the figure-of-eight turns, applying these alternately below and above the elbow. (See Figs. 161, 162.)

F. Complete with one or two circular turns around the lower arm. (See Figs. 163, 164.)

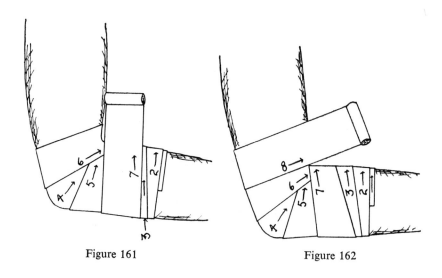

Figure 161

Figure 162

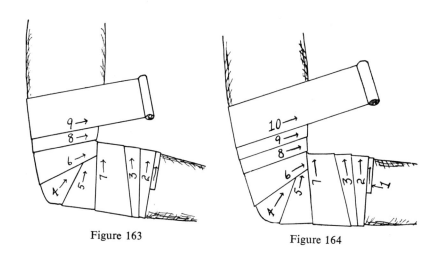

Figure 163

Figure 164

Table III

Bandaging Key for the Upper Extremity

Anatomical Part	Geometric Configuration	Turns	Width of Bandage
1. Wrist	cylinder	circular; spiral	2 in.
2. A. Palm and dorsum of hand	cylinder	circular; spiral	2 in.
B. Palm and wrist	joint	figure-of-eight	2 in.
3. Finger			
(a) Tip	ovoid	recurrent	¾ and 1 in.
(b) Body	cylinder (occasionally cone-shaped)	spiral spiral reverse	¾ and 1 in.
4. A. Thumb			
(a) Tip	ovoid	recurrent	¾ and 1 in.
(b) Body	cylinder or cone	spiral, or spiral reverse	¾ and 1 in.
B. Thumb and wrist	wide part and narrow	figure-of-eight ("spica")	¾ and 1 in.
5. Forearm			
(a) Lower	cylinder	circular and spiral	2 in.
(b) Upper	cone	spiral reverse	2 and 3 in.
6. Arm	cylinder cone	circular, spiral and spiral reverse	2, 2½, 3 in.
7. Elbow			
(a) Extension	cylinder or cone	spiral, or spiral reverse	2, 2½, 3 in.
(b) Flexion	joint	figure-of-eight	3 in.

14

Bandages for the Lower Extremity

1. Anatomico-physiological structure.
2. General principles.
3. Bandaging the lower leg.
4. Bandaging the toes.
5. Bandaging the foot.
6. Bandaging the ankle joint.
7. Bandaging the heel.
8. Bandaging the leg.
9. Bandaging the knee.
10. Bandaging the thigh.

1. ANATOMICO-PHYSIOLOGICAL STRUCTURE

The superficial nerves, veins, and lymphatics of the lower extremity have been presented previously. The muscles and main arteries of the lower extremity are herein presented. (See Figs. 167, 168, 169, 170, 171.)

2. GENERAL PRINCIPLES

The general principles of bandaging the lower extremity are practically identical with those of the upper extremity. The cylinder-shaped portion of the leg just above the ankle joint serves as a starting point for many of the bandages of the lower portion of the lower extremity. Following the application of the anchoring circular turns, one may proceed to the toes, the foot, the ankle joint, or upward upon the leg. The application of firm, anchoring, circular turns to a part as active as the lower extremity, needs little justification.

90

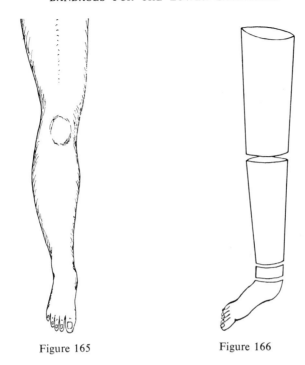

Figure 165   Figure 166

3. BANDAGING THE LOWER LEG (two-, two-and-one-half- and three-inch bandages)

This portion of the leg is a cylinder and is bandaged with simple circular turns. One or more spiral turns may be used to cover an area slightly wider than the width of the bandage. (See Fig. 172.)

4. BANDAGING THE TOES (three-fourths or one-inch bandages)

Each toe consists of two geometric figures. The tip is part of an ovoid and requires recurrent turns. The body is a cylinder and is bandaged with spiral turns. (See *Bandaging of the fingers.*)

A. Anchor the bandage with two circular turns above the ankle. (See Fig. 173.)

B. Carry the roller across the dorsum of the foot to the toe. (See Fig. 174.)

C. Bandage the toe with several ascending spiral turns. (See Fig. 175.)

D. Carry the roller back across the dorsum of the foot. (See Fig. 176.)

E. Fix the bandage with several circular turns around the lower leg. (See Fig. 177.)

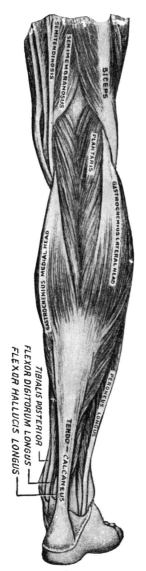

Figure 167
Posterior Muscles of the Leg.

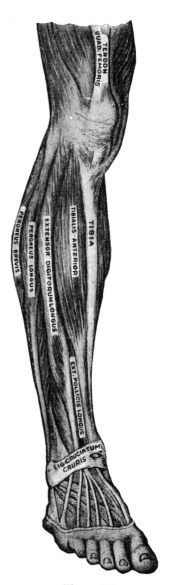

Figure 168
Anterior Muscles of the Leg.

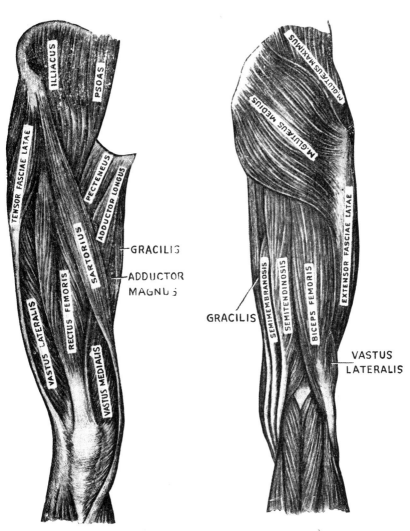

Figure 169
Anterior Thigh Muscles.

Figure 170
Posterior Thigh Muscles.

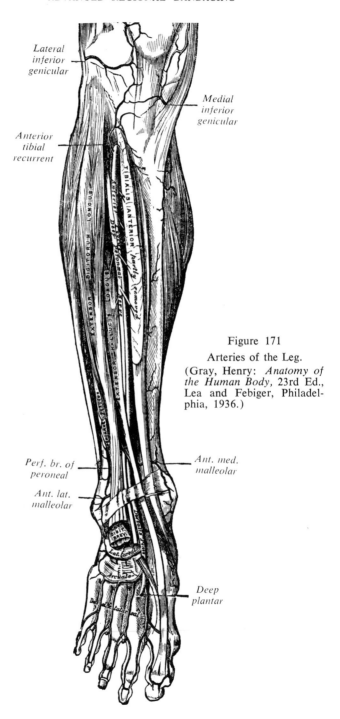

Lateral inferior genicular

Medial inferior genicular

Anterior tibial recurrent

Figure 171

Arteries of the Leg.
(Gray, Henry: *Anatomy of the Human Body,* 23rd Ed., Lea and Febiger, Philadelphia, 1936.)

Perf. br. of peroneal

Ant. med. malleolar

Ant. lat. malleolar

Deep plantar

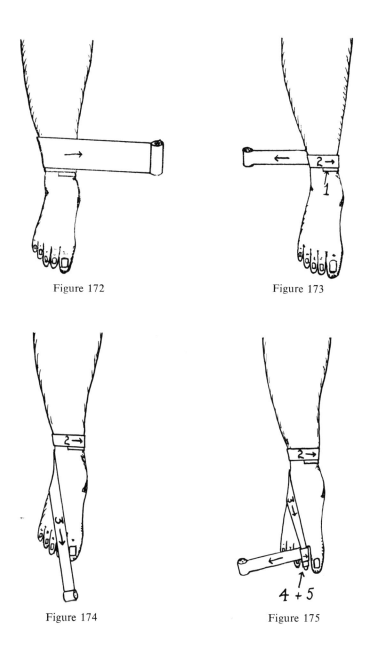

Figure 172

Figure 173

Figure 174

Figure 175

If the tip of the toe is to be included in the bandage, then prior to the application of the ascending spiral in *C* above, apply two or three recurrent turns over the tip of the toe.

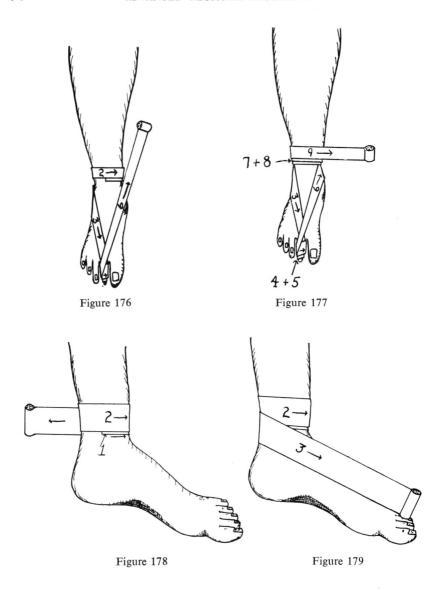

Figure 176   Figure 177

Figure 178   Figure 179

5. BANDAGING THE FOOT (two- and two-and-one-half-inch bandages)

The foot is primarily a cone, although the most distal portion, just proximal to the toes, is cylindrical in shape. Bandages of the foot are anchored at the lower leg. The roller is carried to the most distal portion of the foot, from which it ascends. One or two spiral turns are applied, the spiral reverse is used for several turns, and the roller is then carried to the lower leg, where it is fixed with several circular turns.

The most desirable bandage for the foot, however, is one which is also employed for the ankle joint, namely, the figure-of-eight.

Directions for Figure-of-Eight of the Foot

A. Anchor the bandage with one or two circular turns around the lower leg. (See Fig. 178.)

B. Carry the roller to the distal part of the foot. (See Fig. 179.)

C. Apply two slow ascending spiral turns. (See Figs. 180, 181, 182.)

D. Proceed upward on the foot with a series of ascending figures-of-eight around the foot and ankle joint. (See Figs. 183, 184, 185, 186, 187, 188.)

E. Fix with several circular turns around the lower leg (See Fig. 189.)

6. BANDAGING THE ANKLE JOINT (two- and two-and-one-half-inch bandages)

The ankle joint is best bandaged by a series of ascending figures-of-eight as in the *Figure-of-eight of the Foot,* already described and illustrated. (See previous directions.)

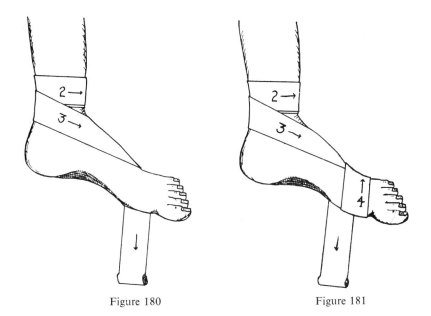

Figure 180   Figure 181

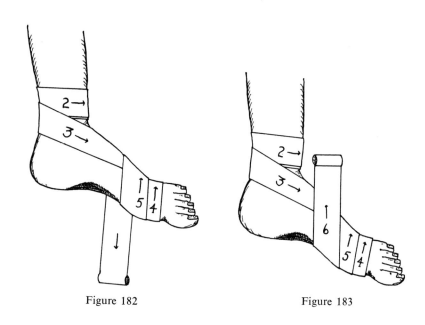

Figure 182   Figure 183

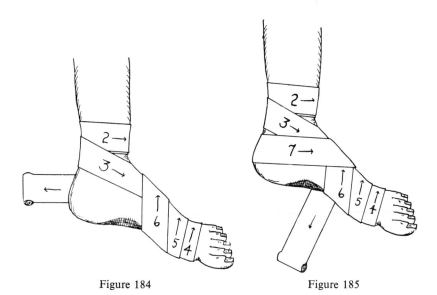

Figure 184   Figure 185

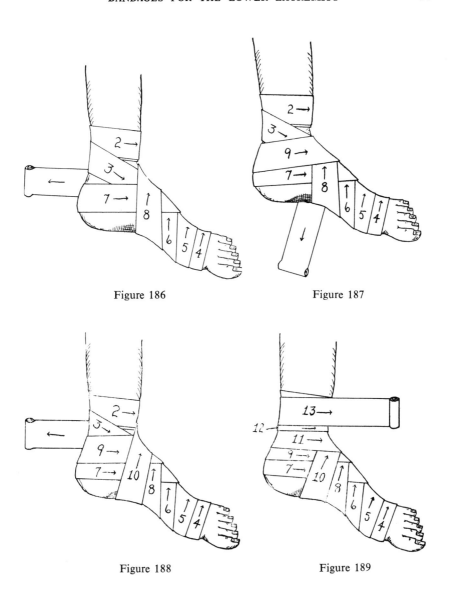

Figure 186

Figure 187

Figure 188

Figure 189

7. BANDAGING THE HEEL (three-inch bandage)

The point of the heel is a rather difficult area to cover; however, figure-of-eight turns best serve the purpose. The point of the heel is covered first and then eccentric or divergent figure-of-eight turns are applied, to hold the first turn in place.

Directions

A. Apply one or two circular turns around the lower leg to anchor the bandage. (See Fig. 190.)

B. Apply a circular turn around the point of the heel. (See Fig. 191.)

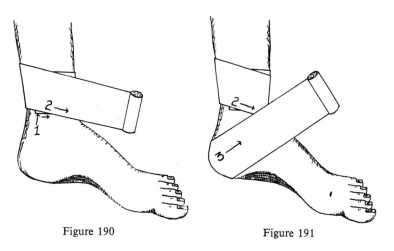

Figure 190   Figure 191

C. Start the first figure-of-eight turn by a loop around the proximal portion of the foot. This turn should overlap the lower border of the circular turn around the point of the heel. (See Fig. 192.)

D. Apply the second loop of the figure-of-eight turn around the lower part of the leg. This turn should overlap the upper border of the circular turn around the heel (See Fig. 193); thus, the first figure-of-eight turn serves to fix the circular turn which covers the point of the heel.

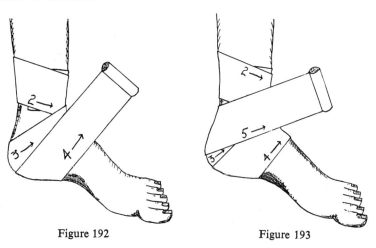

Figure 192   Figure 193

E. Continue the figure-of-eight turns, applying these alternately below and above the heel. (See Figs. 194, 195.)

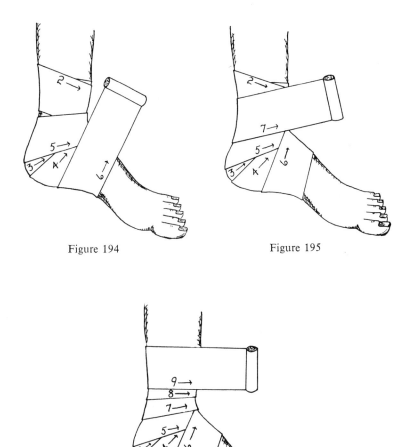

Figure 194   Figure 195

Figure 196

F. Complete with one or two circular turns around the lower leg. (See Fig. 196.)

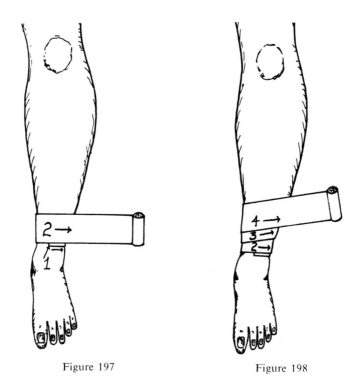

Figure 197   Figure 198

8. BANDAGING THE LEG (two-, two-and-one-half- and three-inch
   bandages)

   The leg consists of a lower cylindrical portion and an upper cone-
shaped portion. The lower part is bandaged with a series of slow ascending spirals, and at the point of transition from cylinder to cone, the spiral
reverse is begun.

Directions

   A. Anchor the bandage with one or two circular turns around the
lower leg. (See Fig. 197.)
   B. With slow ascending spirals, proceed up the leg. (See Fig. 198.)
   C. When the cone-shaped portion is reached, apply spiral reverses
until the leg is covered. (See Figs. 199, 200.)

9. BANDAGING THE KNEE (three-inch bandage)

   The bandages for the knee will vary, depending upon whether it is
kept in the extended position, or in the partly flexed position. If the knee
is at rest, and kept extended, it may be bandaged as are the leg and thigh,

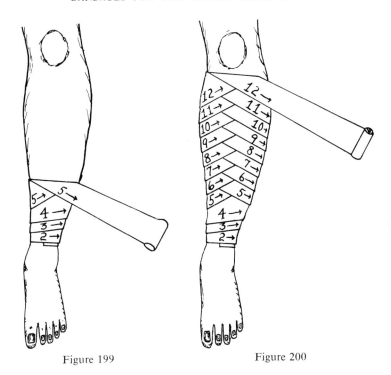

Figure 199   Figure 200

with spiral, or spiral reverses depending upon which of these is more adaptable; however, in bandaging the knee in a position of flexion, the figure-of-eight is used. The knee is first covered with a circular turn and then eccentric figures-of-eight are applied to hold this first turn in place.

Directions

A. Apply one or two circular turns and spiral turns to the upper leg to anchor the bandage. (See Fig. 201.)

B. Apply a circular turn around the point of the knee. (See Fig. 202.)

C. Start the first figure-of-eight turn by a loop around the upper leg. This turn should overlap the lower border of the circular turn around the point of the knee. (See Fig. 203.)

D. Apply the second loop of the figure-of-eight turn around the lower thigh. This turn should overlap the upper border of the circular turn around the knee (See Fig. 204); thus, the first figure-of-eight turn serves to fix the circular turn which covers the point of the knee.

E. Continue the figure-of-eight turns, applying these alternately below and above the knee. (See Figs. 205, 206.)

F. Complete with one or two circular or spiral turns around the lower thigh. (See Fig. 207.)

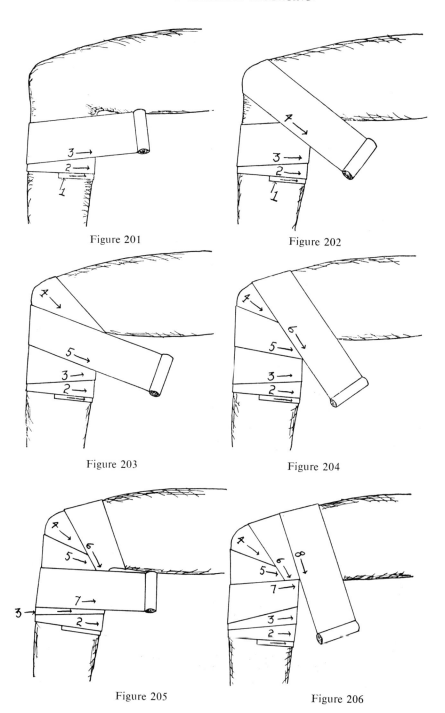

Figure 201

Figure 202

Figure 203

Figure 204

Figure 205

Figure 206

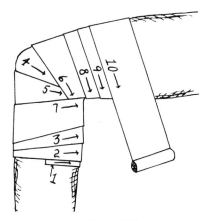

Figure 207

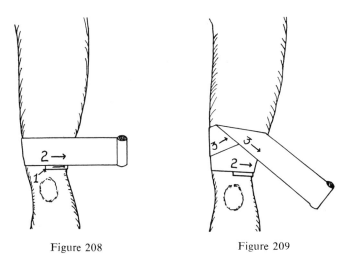

Figure 208   Figure 209

10. BANDAGING THE THIGH (three-inch bandage)

The thigh is a cone and is bandaged with spiral reverse turns.

Directions

A. Apply one or two circular turns, just above the knee, to anchor the bandage. (See Fig. 208.)

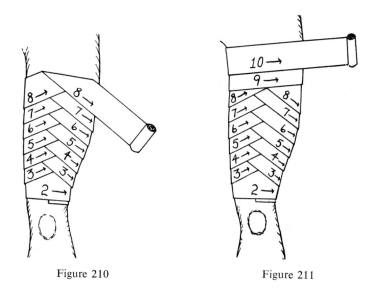

Figure 210   Figure 211

B. Continue with simple spiral and spiral reverse turns until the part is covered. (See Figs. 209, 210.) The choice between spiral and spiral reverse turns will depend upon the configuration of the part.

C. Terminate with one or two circular or spiral turns. (See Fig. 211.)

Table IV

Bandaging Key for the Lower Extremity

Anatomical Part	Geometric Configuration	Turns	Width of Bandage
1. Lower leg (just above ankle joint)	cylinder	circular, spiral	2, 2½, and 3 in.
2. Foot:			
A. Distal part	cylinder	circular, spiral	2 and 2½ in.
B. Proximal part	cone	spiral reverse	2 and 2½ in.
3. Ankle joint (foot and lower leg)	joint	figure-of-eight	2 and 2½ in.
4. Toes:			
A. Tip	part of ovoid	recurrent	¾ or 1 in.
B. Body	cylinder	spiral	¾ or 1 in.
5. Heel	joint	figure-of-eight	3 in.
6. Leg			
A. Lower part	cylinder	circular and spiral	2, 2½, and 3 in.
B. Upper part	cone	spiral reverse	2, 2½, and 3 in.
7. Knee			
A. Extension	cylinder or cone	spiral or spiral reverse	3 in.
B. Flexion	joint	figure-of-eight	3 in.
8. Thigh	cylinder, cone	circular spiral and spiral reverse	3 in.

15

Bandages for the Head, Face, and Neck

1. Anatomico-physiological structure.
2. General considerations.
3. Bandaging the neck.
4. Bandaging the neck and head.
5. Bandaging the scalp.
6. Bandaging the eyes, ears, and mastoids.
7. Four-tailed binder for lower jaw.
8. The Barton bandage.

1. ANATOMICO-PHYSIOLOGICAL STRUCTURE

The head, face, and neck present a series of anatomico-physiological factors which are of considerable significance when one is confronted with bandaging any of these parts. Bandages and surgical dressings over these parts must not interfere with the functioning of the eyes, ears, nose, or mouth, unless these are the involved parts. A bandage for an injury of the scalp must not be so tightened under the chin as to interfere with the proper chewing of food. The face and the organs concerned with the special senses are particularly sensitive structures and thus one should make an attempt to apply dressings over these areas with extreme care and patience. Excessive tightness, or pressure, interferes considerably with the comfort of the patient.

108

2. GENERAL CONSIDERATIONS

The head is an ovoid, and as was stressed in an earlier chapter, proper fixation is the keynote to successful bandaging of this type of figure. The anchoring circular turns, for bandages of the head, may be applied in two main directions: (a) Vertically, from the vertex or top of the head, around the face to the chin; and (b) horizontally, around the vault of the cranium from the occiput to the forehead.

The chin and the occiput serve as two excellent anchoring points, off which the bandage will not slip.

An important principle in bandages about the head is best illustrated by the method employed in tying a package. In the box illustrated below, a circular turn is first applied about the center. (See Fig. 212.) At the completion of the circular turn, the two ends are locked and these then diverge from each other to encircle the long diameter of the box. These ends are then tied where they meet again. (See Fig. 213.) In a similar fashion, these "package turns" may be applied to the head. These turns serve as a general utility bandage to hold dressings in place over most parts of the scalp, face, chin, and possibly the ears. These turns also serve to indicate the two main directions and courses of the vertical and horizontal anchoring turns used in most bandages of the head. (See Figs. 214, 215, 216.)

3. BANDAGING THE NECK (two-inch bandage)

The neck is a cylinder and is bandaged with one or two circular turns. If necessary, one or two spiral turns may be applied. (See Fig. 217.)

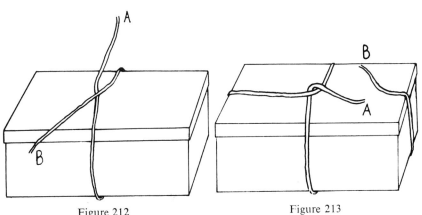

Figure 212   Figure 213

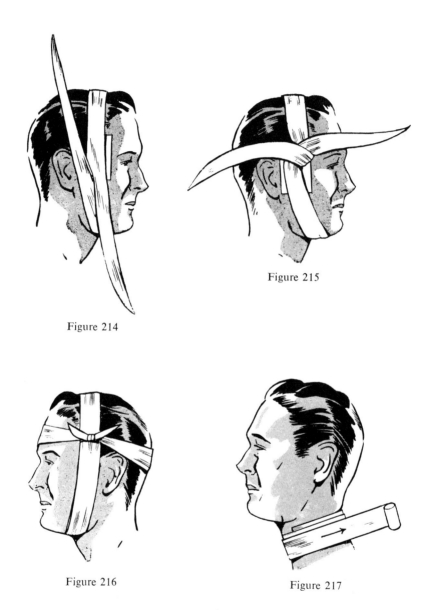

Figure 214

Figure 215

Figure 216

Figure 217

4. BANDAGING THE NECK AND HEAD (two-inch bandage)

Occasionally, the necessity arises for holding a large dressing in place over the back of the neck and lower part of the head. The "Figure-of-eight of the Head and Neck" serves this purpose well.

Directions

A. Apply one or two circular turns around the neck. (See Fig. 218.)

B. Carry the bandage upward on the back of the neck, and, passing just beneath the occiput, carry the bandage around the head, above the opposite ear. (See Fig. 219.)

C. Bring the roller across the forehead, and around the head over the proximal ear and around the neck. (See Fig. 220.) This completes the first figure-of-eight.

D. Carry the roller around the neck, and then around the head to complete the second figure-of-eight. (See Fig. 221.) This may be repeated with as many turns as are necessary to adequately cover the part.

E. Terminate with one to two circular turns around the neck.

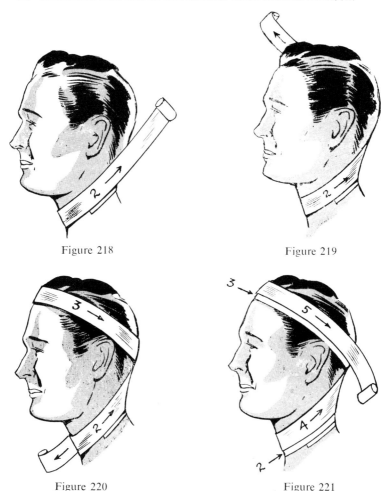

Figure 218   Figure 219

Figure 220   Figure 221

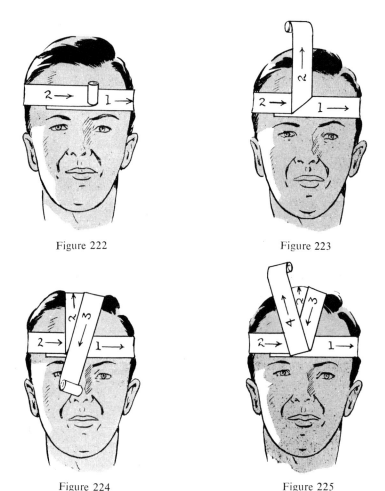

Figure 222

Figure 223

Figure 224

Figure 225

5. BANDAGING THE SCALP (two- and three-inch bandages)

The head is an ovoid and thus to bandage the scalp one must employ recurrent turns. The anchoring circular turns are applied across the forehead, around the side of the head, above the ear, under the occiput, and around the other side of the head, above the ear, and back to the forehead. One or two of these turns may be applied for anchoring the bandage. Sufficient recurrent turns are then applied to cover the scalp either partly or completely. Terminate with one to two circular turns around the forehead. (For the method of application of these recurrent turns, see Unit II, Chapter 8, *Bandaging of Ovoids.*) (See Figs. 222, 223, 224, 225, 226, 227.)

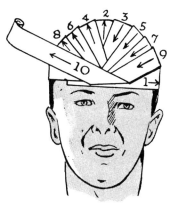

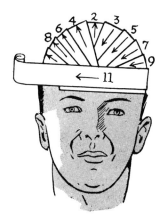

Figure 226   Figure 227

It will be noted that in the application of the recurrent turns as above described and illustrated, it is necessary for either the patient, or an assistant, to hold each turn in place until the final fixing circular turns are applied. To eliminate the necessity for assistance, one may use a double roller, consisting of a two-inch bandage and a three-inch bandage. The principle of application here is that each recurrent turn is anchored by a circular turn, the three-inch bandage serving for the recurrent turns and the two-inch bandage for the circular turns. This bandage is known as the "capeline of the head."

6. BANDAGING THE EYES, EARS, AND MASTOIDS (two-inch bandage)

The eyes, ears, and mastoids are bandaged by a series of circular and spiral turns. These turns differ from other circular turns around the head in that they are applied in an oblique fashion. The basic principle in both is essentially the same, namely, to have the circular turns pass under the occiput. This prevents the bandage from slipping off the top of the head. After initial fixation of the bandage with one or two horizontal circular turns around the forehead and under the occiput, the bandage may be used to cover the eyes, ears, or mastoids. These circular turns deviate or tilt in any desired direction. A downward tilting of the turns on one side of the head is compensated for by an upward tilting over the opposite side of the head.

Bandaging the Eye

1. Apply a circular turn around the forehead and occiput. (See Fig. 228.)

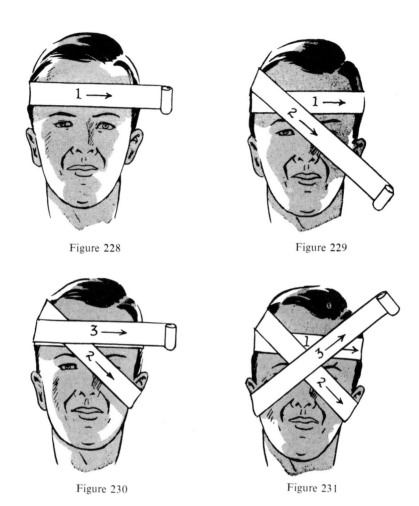

Figure 228   Figure 229

Figure 230   Figure 231

2. Apply an oblique circular turn covering the eye. (See Fig. 229.)

3. Fix the oblique turn with a second circular turn, similar to the first. (See Fig. 230.)

4. Apply alternating oblique and horizontal turns until the eye is adequately covered.

Bandaging Both Eyes

1. Apply a circular turn around the forehead and occiput. (See Fig. 228.)

2. Apply an oblique circular turn covering one eye. (See Fig. 229.)

3. Instead of repeating the horizontal turn around the forehead as in the bandage for one eye (See Fig. 230), carry the roller around

under the occiput, and apply an oblique circular turn which covers the opposite eye. (See Fig. 231.) Continue to apply alternating oblique circular turns first to one eye and then the other until both are adequately covered.

4. Terminate with one or two circular turns around the forehead.

Bandaging the Ear and Mastoid

1. Apply a horizontal circular turn around the forehead and occiput. (See Fig. 232.)

2. Apply an oblique circular turn covering the lower part of the ear. (See Fig. 233.)

3. Apply a series of oblique circular turns, each ascending slightly and partly overlapping the previous turn. (See Fig. 234.)

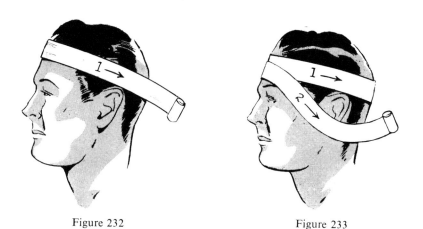

Figure 232   Figure 233

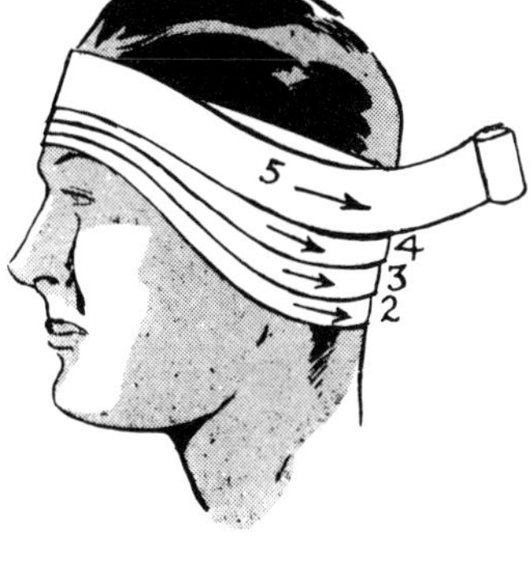

Figure 234

7. FOUR-TAILED BINDER FOR LOWER JAW

This is an excellent dressing for immobilization and splinting of the lower jaw. The body of the binder is placed under the chin. The two upper tails are carried around the face horizontally and tied to each other under the occiput. The two lower tails are carried vertically and tied to each other over the vertex of the skull. (See Figs. 235, 236.)

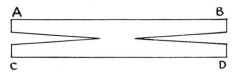

Figure 235

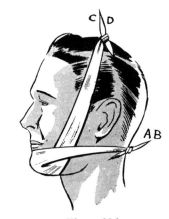

Figure 236

8. THE BARTON BANDAGE FOR THE JAW

This is a bandage used by many surgical dressers for immobilization and splinting of the lower jaw following fractures of the mandible. It consists of vertical turns which pass over the top of the head and pass under the chin, and also of horizontal turns which are applied anteriorly over the chin and posteriorly around the back of the neck. A careful analysis of this bandage reveals that the horizontal turns around the front of the chin tend to pull the lower jaw backward, and thereby increase the displacement in certain types of fractures. It is recommended that the simple "package turns," described previously, be used for immobilization in fractures, or injuries of the mandible. It is the vertical turns of the latter which serve to splint the mandible against the maxilla, or upper jaw.

16

Bandages for the Neck, Chest, and Axilla

1. General principles.
2. Bandaging the neck.
3. Bandaging the neck and one axilla.
4. Bandaging the neck and both axillae.
5. Bandaging the neck and chest.

1. GENERAL PRINCIPLES

The neck, chest, and axillae present an anatomical structure which allows for the application of a wide variety of the basic turns alone, or in combination. Which of these is applied in any particular case will depend on the exact location of the area to be covered. In children, or in those patients who are likely to move the dressing, it is advisable to apply the more secure type of bandages. Thus a figure-of-eight around two parts would be more secure than a simple circular turn around one part.

2. BANDAGING THE NECK (two-, two-and-one-half-, and three-inch bandages)

The neck is a cylinder and is bandaged with several circular turns or spiral turns. (See Fig. 217.) These circular turns may also serve as anchoring turns for the more complex bandages to follow.

3. BANDAGING THE NECK AND ONE AXILLA (two-, two-and-one-half-, and three-inch bandages)

The neck and axilla are two relatively remote structures and are best bandaged with a series of figure-of-eight turns.

Directions

A. Apply one or two circular turns around the neck to anchor the bandage. (See Fig. 237.)

B. Carry the bandage across the front of the shoulder and under the axilla. This completes the first loop of the figure-of-eight turn. (See Fig. 238.)

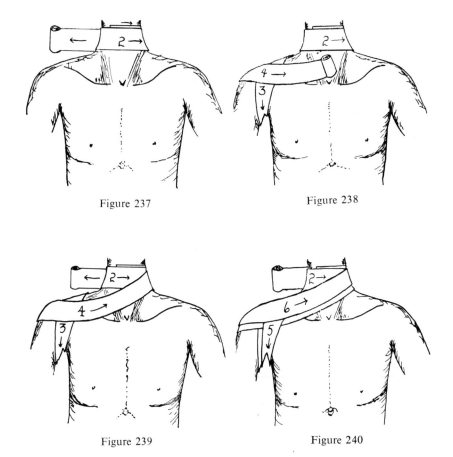

Figure 237

Figure 238

Figure 239

Figure 240

C. Carry the roller across the front of the neck and apply the second loop of the figure-of-eight by a turn around the neck. This completes the first figure-of-eight turn. (See Fig. 239.)

D. Repeat with as many figure-of-eight turns as are necessary to adequately cover the part. (See Fig. 240.)

E. Terminate with one or two circular turns around the neck. (See Fig. 241.)

4. BANDAGING THE NECK AND BOTH AXILLAE (two-, two-and-one-half-, and three-inch bandages)

This bandage is similar to the previous one, except that at the completion of the first figure-of-eight turn (See Fig. 239), instead of returning to the same axilla for a second turn, the bandage is carried to the opposite axilla and a figure-of-eight turn is applied around this axilla and the neck. (See Fig. 242.) A second figure-of-eight is then applied to the neck and first axilla. In this manner alternate figure-of-eight turns are applied, passing first around one axilla and the neck, and then around the second axilla and the neck; thus, this constitutes a double figure-of-eight of the neck and both axillae, or "Double Spica of Neck and Axillae."

5. BANDAGING THE NECK AND CHEST (two-, two-and-one-half-, and three-inch bandages)

This bandage is particularly valuable for maintaining dressings in place over the upper chest and the lower part of the neck, near their junction. It is the "Figure-of-eight of the Neck and Chest."

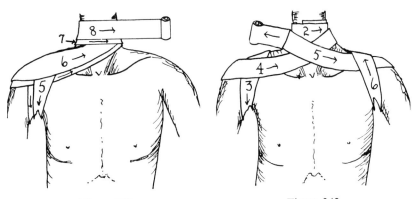

Figure 241   Figure 242

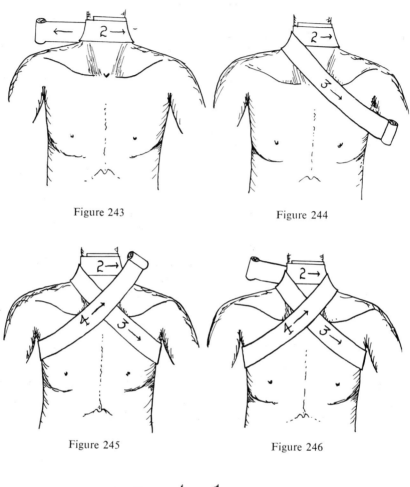

Figure 243

Figure 244

Figure 245

Figure 246

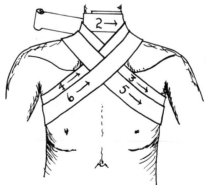

Figure 247

Directions

A. Apply one or two circular turns around the neck to anchor the bandage. (See Fig. 243.)

B. Carry the bandage across the upper part of the chest to the opposite axilla. (See Fig. 244.)

C. Carry the bandage across the back and around under the other axilla. (See Fig. 245.) This completes the first loop of the figure-of-eight.

D. Return to the neck and apply a circular turn around the neck, thereby completing the first figure-of-eight turn. (See Fig. 246.)

E. Repeat with as many figure-of-eight turns as are necessary to cover the part. (See Fig. 247.)

17

Bandages for the Chest and Abdomen

1. Anatomico-physiological structure.
2. General principles.
3. Bandaging the chest.
4. Bandaging the abdomen.
5. Many-tailed binder or Scultetus bandage.

1. ANATOMICO-PHYSIOLOGICAL STRUCTURE

Although the average chest and abdomen resemble the cylinder in contour, occasionally, and particularly as a result of the development of special muscles, the contour may more closely resemble a cone. For the most part, however, there is moderate uniformity in the general outline of the chest and abdomen. The muscular structure of these is herein demonstrated. (See Figs. 248, 249.)

2. GENERAL PRINCIPLES

A variety of bandages may be applied to the chest and abdomen, the particular type of turn depending on the contour of the parts and the degree of muscular development. Most commonly cylindrical in shape, these may be bandaged with circular and spiral turns. For the cone-shaped trunk, the spiral reverse may be used. These turns may be applied as either ascending or descending bandages.

3. BANDAGING THE CHEST (four-, five-, and six-inch bandages)

The descending bandages are usually preferable for bandaging the chest.

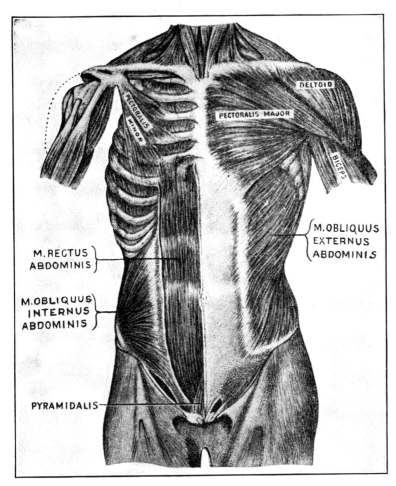

Figure 248. Muscles of the Chest and Abdominal Wall.

Directions

A. Apply one or two circular turns to anchor the bandage. (See Fig. 250.) These should pass around the upper part of the chest, just under the axilla. It is advisable to place some padding material in the axilla to protect the delicate skin.

B. Apply a series of descending spiral turns until the part is adequately covered. (See Fig. 251.) If the chest is cone-shaped, apply descending spiral reverses.

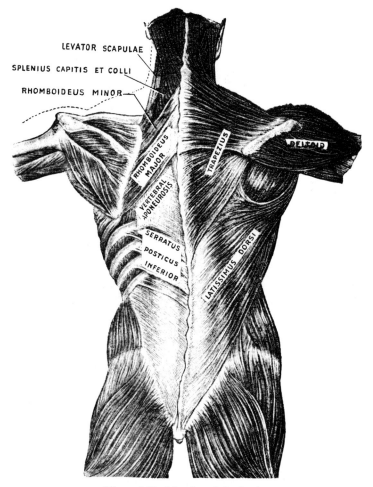

Figure 249. Muscles of the Back.

4. BANDAGING THE ABDOMEN (four-, five-, and six-inch bandages)

The abdomen is bandaged in a fashion similar to that used in bandaging the chest. Being cylindrical in shape, it is covered with circular and spiral turns.

Directions

A. Apply one or two circular turns to anchor the bandage. (See Fig. 252.)

B. Apply several descending spiral turns until the part is adequately covered. (See Fig. 253.)

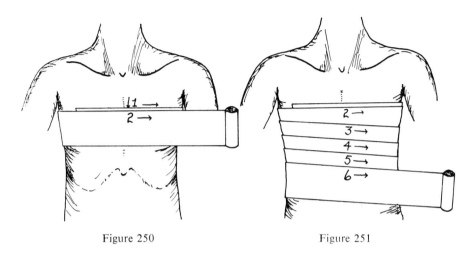

Figure 250

Figure 251

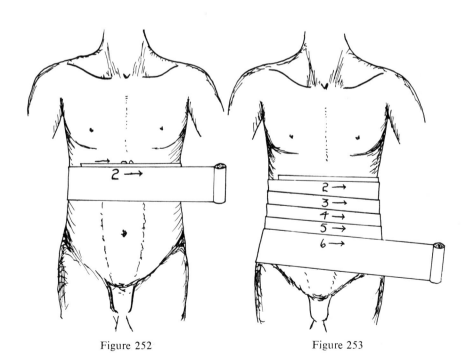

Figure 252

Figure 253

5. MANY-TAILED BINDER OR SCULTETUS BANDAGE

Occasionally, it becomes necessary to apply an abdominal bandage to a patient who is lying in bed. It would be a difficult task to raise the patient each time the roller had to be carried across the back. In addition, the patient may not be able to tolerate such manipulation. To obviate this, and to obtain good support of the abdomen, the many-tailed binder or Scultetus bandage is used.

SCULTETUS: Johannis Sculteti (1595-1645), called Scultetus, was famous for his illustrations of surgical procedures and various surgical instruments. His *Armamentarium Chirurgicum,* published in 1653, presents an interesting sidelight on the various operations of the time. These are demonstrated in a series of excellent plates showing such procedures as amputation of the breast, reduction of dislocations, passage of sounds, forceps delivery, and many others. The following illustrations show the original many-tailed binder as applied by Scultetus to the thigh and leg. (See Figs. 254, 255.)

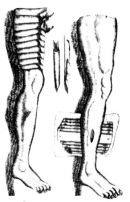

Figures 254 and 255

The binder consists primarily of a large flat piece of material, the lateral borders of which consist of numerous strips or tails. The binder may also be prepared by sewing several strips of roller bandage together, each overlapping the next, in a shingle fashion. These are attached along the middle one quarter of the strips, leaving the ends free. (See Fig. 256.)

Directions

Assume the patient is lying on his or her back in bed.

A. Pass one border of the binder beneath the back of the patient so that there is a border with its tails on each side of the patient. (See Fig. 257.)

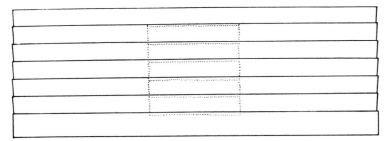

Figure 256

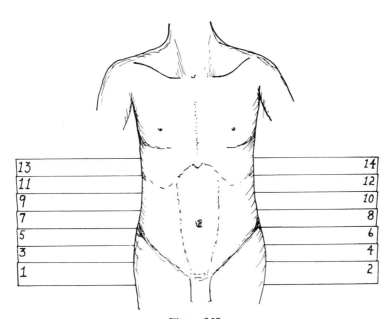

Figure 257

B. Carry the lowest end or tail on one border across the abdomen in a diagonally upward direction. (See Fig. 258.)

C. Carry the lowest tail of the opposite border across the abdomen in a diagonally upward direction, thereby partly overlapping the first end. (See Fig. 259.)

D. Carry the next tail of the first border across the abdomen. This overlaps both tails No. 1 and No. 2.

E. Continue to carry alternate tails across the abdomen, in an ascending fashion, until all have been applied. (See Fig. 260.) Pin these in place with a series of vertically applied safety pins. (See Fig. 261.)

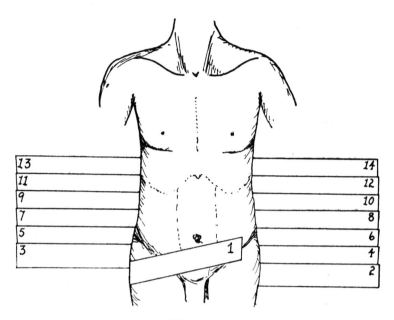

Figure 258

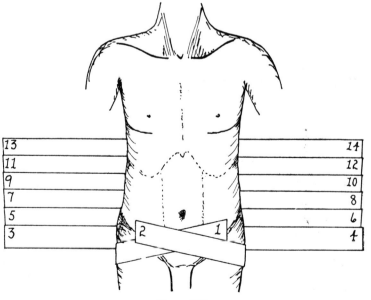

Figure 259

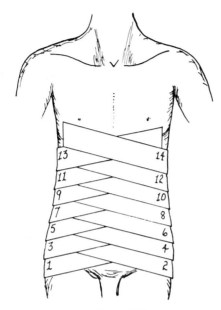

Figure 260

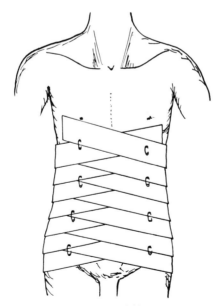

Figure 261

With the Scultetus or many-tailed binder it is possible to obtain considerable pressure and support with the overlapping turns.

18

Bandages for the Breasts

1. General principles.
2. Bandage for the breast, shoulder, and chest ("spica of breast").
3. Bandage for both breasts ("double spica of breasts").
4. Double-T binder for breasts.

1. GENERAL PRINCIPLES

The breasts, because of their location, allow for the application of a variety of turns. The primary objectives in bandaging a breast may be threefold, namely: (a) To hold dressings in place; (b) to lift and support the breast; (c) to compress the breast against the chest wall.

In supporting and compressing a breast, the ideal direction for lifting it is toward the opposite shoulder; thus, most bandages of the breast include turns around the opposite shoulder. In all breast bandages, it is preferable to have the bandage applied over the breast first, and then over the shoulder; thus, as the roller is being carried from the breast to the shoulder, an upward pull can be exerted upon the breast.

2. BANDAGE FOR THE BREAST, SHOULDER, AND THORAX
(Spica of Breast) (three- and four-inch bandages)

This is the most commonly used bandage for both lifting and compressing the breast. It consists of a series of figure-of-eight turns, each consisting of one loop around the affected breast and the opposite

130

shoulder, and the other loop around the thorax. These are applied in an ascending manner. This bandage is sometimes referred to as the "Suspensory of the Breast."

Directions

A. Beginning under the affected breast, apply a circular turn around the chest by carrying the roller across the front of the chest, under the uninvolved breast, and around the back to the starting point. (See Fig. 262.) A second circular turn should be applied to firmly anchor the bandage. This completes the first loop of the figure-of-eight.

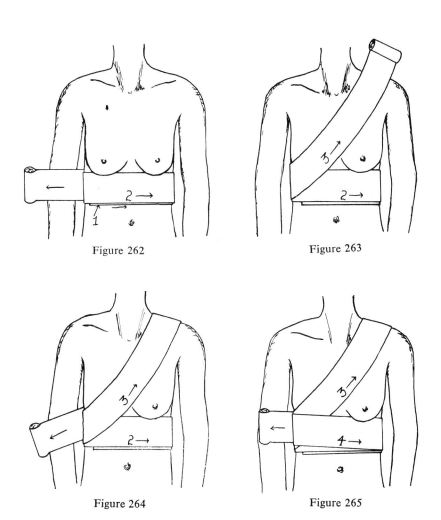

Figure 262   Figure 263

Figure 264   Figure 265

B. Carry the bandage under the affected breast and over the opposite shoulder. (See Fig. 263.)

C. Return to the starting point by carrying the roller diagonally across the back. (See Fig. 264.) This completes the second loop of the figure-of-eight turn.

D. The next turn is a circular turn around the chest, similar to the first, but slightly above and overlapping it. (See Fig. 265.)

E. The second figure-of-eight is completed by a second turn around the breast and opposite shoulder, but slightly above and partly overlapping the first turn. (See Fig. 266.) This completes the second figure-of-eight turn.

F. Apply these ascending alternate turns around the thorax and the breast and shoulder, until the entire breast is adequately covered. (See Fig. 267.)

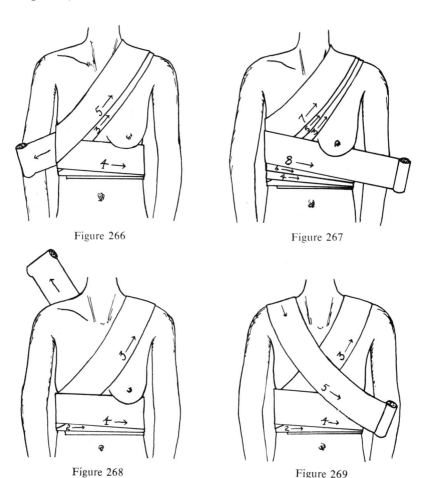

Figure 266   Figure 267

Figure 268   Figure 269

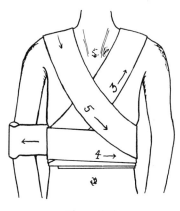

Figure 270

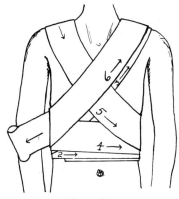

Figure 271

3. BANDAGE FOR BOTH BREASTS (*Double Spica of the Breasts*) (three- and four-inch bandages)

This bandage is similar to the above bandage for one breast, except that figure-of-eight turns are applied around both breasts and their respective opposite shoulders.

Directions

A. Apply a figure-of-eight turn around one breast and the thorax as in the previous bandage. (See Figs. 262, 263, 264.)

B. Carry the roller across the front of the chest, and then diagonally across the back to the opposite shoulder. (See Fig. 268.)

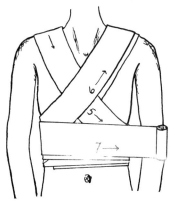

Figure 272

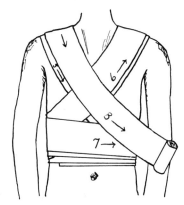

Figure 273

C. Carry the roller downward over the shoulder and over the lower part of the opposite breast. (See Fig. 269.)

D. Carry the roller around the back and repeat the figure-of-eight over the first breast. (See Figs. 270, 271.)

E. Apply a second figure-of-eight to the second breast as previously. (See Figs. 272, 273.)

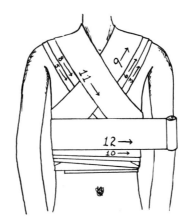

Figure 274

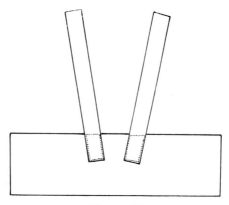

Figure 275

F. Continue with figure-of-eight turns, alternating the breasts, until both are adequately covered. (See Fig. 274.)

4. DOUBLE-"T" BINDER FOR THE BREASTS (eight-inch wide strip; two two-inch strips)

This bandage is especially valuable for the support of the breasts in nursing women, since it is easily removed and reapplied. (See Fig. 275.)

Directions

A. Apply the wide part of the binder to the upper part of the back. (See Fig. 276.)

B. Bring the two wide ends under the axillae, across the front of the breasts; fix these firmly and pin in place. (See Fig. 277.)

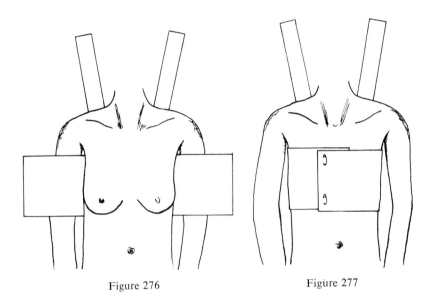

Figure 276   Figure 277

C. Carry the two narrow strips over the shoulders and pin these to the already pinned wide part. (See Fig. 278.)

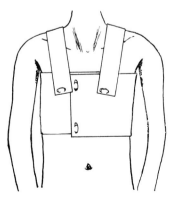

Figure 278

19

Bandages for the Arm, Chest, and Shoulder

1. General principles.
2. Bandaging the shoulder ("spica of the shoulder").
3. Velpeau bandage.
4. Livingston bandage for shoulder and thorax.

1. GENERAL PRINCIPLES

There is a wide variety of bandages which are applicable to the arms, shoulders, and thorax. The individual structure and components of these bandages depend upon the exact parts to be covered as well as the particular positions in which the arm and forearm are to be maintained. Some of these have for their main purpose the mere covering and protection of the parts, while others are applied for immobilization and maintenance of the arm and forearm in certain positions. Included in this group are several of the most commonly used eponymic bandages such as the Velpeau and Livingston bandages.

2. BANDAGING THE SHOULDER (*Spica of the Shoulder*) (three-inch bandage)

This bandage, as its name implies, consists of a series of figure-of-eight turns with loops around the upper arm and chest, with the points of crossing over the affected shoulder.

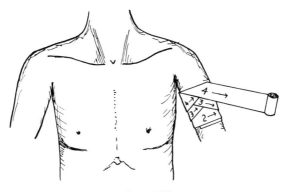

Figure 279

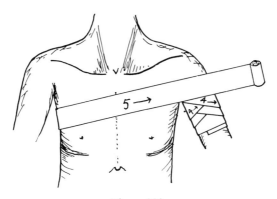

Figure 280

Directions

A. Apply two or three circular and ascending spiral reverse turns over the middle of the arm of the affected side. (See Fig. 279.) These serve to anchor the bandage.

B. Carry the bandage across the upper aspect of the back, under the opposite axilla, and back across the upper anterior chest to the upper part of the bandage on the arm. (See Fig. 280.) This completes the first loop of the figure-of-eight turn.

C. Carry the roller around the arm, ascending at the same time. (See Fig. 281.) This completes the second loop of the figure-of-eight.

D. Continue to apply turns around the chest and arm, in an ascending fashion, until the entire shoulder is covered. (See Figs. 282, 283, 284.)

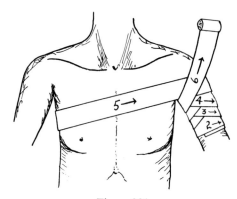

Figure 281

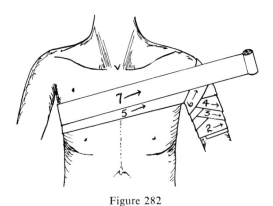

Figure 282

3. VELPEAU BANDAGE

One of the most widely used dressings for injuries around the shoulder joint is the Velpeau bandage. The primary function of this bandage is to immobilize the arm and forearm in a position of flexion across the front of the chest.

VELPEAU: Alfred-Armand-Louis-Marie Velpeau (1795-1867) was originally a blacksmith, an apprentice to his father. He gave this up to study medicine. At the age of 33, he was appointed Surgeon to the Hospital St. Antoine, and later to La Pitié and the Charity Hospital. In 1834, he was made Professor of Clinical Surgery at the Paris Faculty.

Velpeau was not regarded as a scientific worker, but rather as a strong, capable, hard-working teacher and operator. Of Velpeau, Oliver Wendell Holmes once said:

"A good sound head over a pair of wooden shoes is a good deal better than a wooden head belonging to an owner who cases his feet in calf-skin."

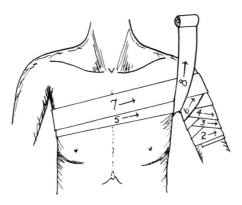

Figure 283

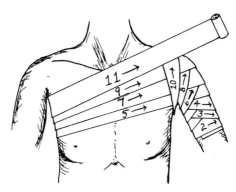

Figure 284

His principal works include his *Treatise on Surgical Anat·omy* (1823), the first detailed work of its kind; his three-volume treatise on operative surgery with atlas (1832), important for its historic data, and once edited in translation by Valentine Mott (1847); and his great treatise on diseases of the breast (1854), the most important work on the subject in its time.

As stated above, the Velpeau bandage is extensively used for a variety of injuries involving the humerus, clavicle, and scapula. It is interesting to note the large number of variations from the original Velpeau bandage; in fact most of the "Velpeau bandages" applied would probably never be recognized by the originator. Herein is included the original description of the Velpeau bandage. (See Fig. 286.)

"But I have contrived a bandage, by means of a simple band, which is adapted both to sternoclavicular luxations, for which I had first designed it, and also to acromioclavicular luxations, fractures of the clavicle, acromion, and scapula and even to fractures of the neck of the humerus. For this purpose we procure a bandage of eight to ten yards in length. The head of this bandage is first applied under the armpit of the sound side, or behind; it is then passed diagonally upon the back and shoulder to the clavicle, upon the side affected. The

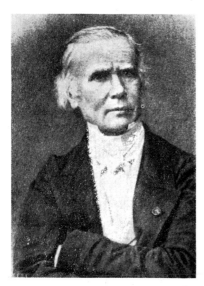

Figure 285. Velpeau.

(Garrison: *Introduction to the History of Medicine,* 4th Ed., W. B. Saunders Co., Philadelphia, 1929.)

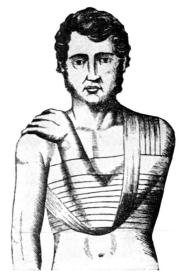

Figure 286.
Velpeau Bandage.

hand of the patient is then placed upon the acromion of the sound shoulder, as if embracing the last. The elbow thus raised is brought in front of the point of the sternum and the affected shoulder is pushed upward, backward, and outward, by the action of the humerus, which, taking its *point d'appui* on the side of the chest, acts like a lever of the first kind, or by a swinglike motion. While an assistant keeps the parts in place, the surgeon brings down the bandage upon the anterior surface of the arm, then outside and under the elbow, to bring it upward and forward under the sound armpit. He repeats this three or four times in order to have that number of diagonal turns, which obliquely traverse the wounded clavicle, the upper part of the chest, and the middle portion of the arm. In place of bringing back the bandage to the affected shoulder, it is afterwards passed horizontally upon the posterior surface of the thorax, and brought back upon the external surface of the arm, elbow, or forearm, in the form of circulars, which are repeated until the hand alone, which is on the sound shoulder, and the stump of the affected one alone remain uncovered. We finish by one or two diagonals, and by a similar number of horizontal circulars. It is unnecessary to add that some paddings and thick compresses may be placed under it in the supraclavicular region, sometimes nearer the sternum, at other times nearer the acromion, according as it seems proper to make pressure on one point rather than another. It is well, also, in order to avoid excoriations of the skin, to place a piece of linen folded double between the chest and arm; and it will be also necessary to adjust a kind of wedge into the armpit, if it is a case of fracture of the neck of the humerus."

Directions

A. Place the arm and forearm of the affected side in such position across the front of the chest so that the hand rests on the opposite shoulder, and the elbow rests in front of and above the lower part of the sternum. Begin the bandage under the axilla of the sound side and carry it across the upper part of the back to the opposite shoulder. (See Fig. 287.)

B. Carry the roller down over the front of the lateral part of the shoulder, down across the middle of the arm, around the arm, and across the front of the chest, back to the starting point under the sound axilla. (See Fig. 288.) This is simply a circular turn around the axilla, shoulder, and arm.

C. Repeat this turn two or three more times, each turn only partly overlapping the previous one. (See Fig. 289.)

D. Carry the bandage across the upper back, in a horizontal fashion, and encircle the arm and anterior chest, to return to the sound axilla. (See Fig. 290.) This is simply a circular turn around the chest and arm.

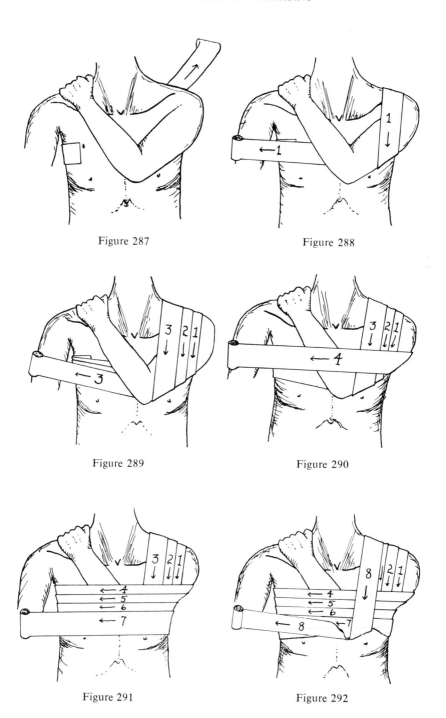

Figure 287

Figure 288

Figure 289

Figure 290

Figure 291

Figure 292

E. Repeat this latter turn, around the chest and arm, several times, each turn only partly overlapping the previous one. (See Fig. 291.)

F. Complete the bandage with one or two more diagonal turns around the shoulder. (See Fig. 292.) One or two more circular turns may then be applied to further fix the bandage.

4. LIVINGSTON'S BANDAGE FOR THE SHOULDER AND THORAX (two- or three-inch bandages)

This is a general utility bandage for either one or both shoulders, and for the upper chest. It combines three of the basic turns, namely: (a) Descending spiral turns over the chest; (b) recurrent turns over one or both shoulders; (c) figure-of-eight turn around the chest, shoulder, and axilla.

This bandage is applied with two rollers of bandage.

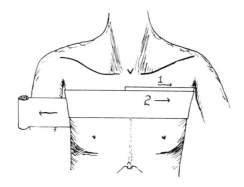

Figure 293

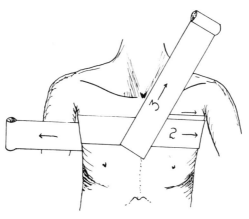

Figure 294

Directions

Roller No. 1 will be used for the spiral turns around the chest. Roller No. 2 will be used for the recurrent turns around the shoulder. Either roller No. 1 or No. 2 may be used for the final figure-of-eight turn.

A. Begin roller No. 1 over the upper part of the sternum and apply one or two circular turns around the chest. (See Fig. 293.)

B. Begin roller No. 2 over the upper part of the sternum, and carry it obliquely upward to the base of the neck on the affected side. (See Fig. 294.)

C. Fix the initial extremity of roller No. 2 by continuing roller No. 1 across the front of the chest. (See Fig. 295.)

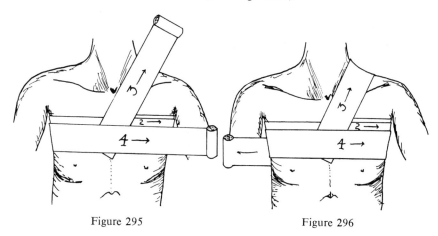

Figure 295   Figure 296

D. Carry roller No. 2 over the shoulder and obliquely downward across the back to a point opposite the starting point. At this point the turn should be caught and held in place by the next turn of roller No. 1. (See Fig. 296.)

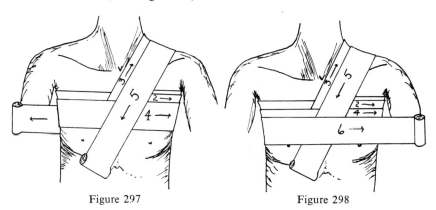

Figure 297   Figure 298

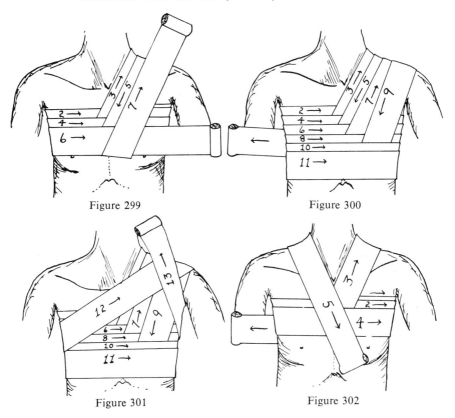

Figure 299   Figure 300

Figure 301   Figure 302

E. Bring roller No. 2 anteriorly, but slightly lateral to, and partly overlapping, the first recurrent turn over the shoulder. (See Fig. 297.)

F. Fix this recurrent turn of roller No. 2 by a spiral turn of roller No. 1, across the chest. (See Fig. 298.)

G. Continue with descending spiral turns of the thorax with roller No. 1, catching both anteriorly and posteriorly the recurrent turns of roller No. 2 over the shoulder. The recurrent turns proceed laterally until the entire shoulder is covered. (See Figs. 299, 300.)

H. To finish the bandage, using either roller No. 1 or roller No. 2, apply a figure-of-eight turn around the affected shoulder and opposite axilla. This serves to prevent slipping of the recurrent turns. (See Fig. 301.)

This bandage may also be applied to both shoulders. The principles are essentially the same, except that following the first turn over the shoulder, the bandage, instead of being carried back over the same shoulder, is carried anteriorly around the opposite shoulder. (See Fig. 302.) The oblique turns of roller No. 2 are maintained in place by repeated descending spiral turns of roller No. 1. Thus roller No. 2 is carried

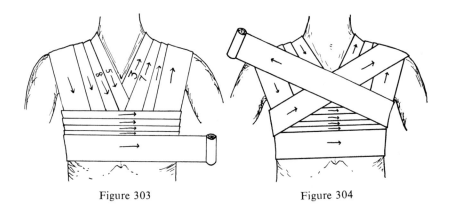

Figure 303   Figure 304

alternately over one shoulder and then the next; thus it travels from anterior to posterior over the left shoulder, and from posterior to anterior over the right shoulder. To complete the bandage, a figure-of-eight turn is applied over both axillae and shoulders. (See Figs. 303, 304.)

20

Bandages for
the Groin, Perineum, and Buttock

1. General principles.
2. Bandaging the groin and upper thigh.
3. Bandaging both groins.
4. Bandaging the buttock.
5. Bandaging the perineum.

1. GENERAL PRINCIPLES

The groin, perineum, and buttocks are bandaged by the simple application of the basic principles previously described. The groin, which is the point of junction of a wide part, the lower abdomen, and a narrow part, the thigh, is best bandaged by a series of figure-of-eight turns. Similar turns may be utilized to cover the buttocks as well as the lateral aspect of the upper thigh. The perineum may be dressed with the basic turns; however, the most practical dressing for this region is the T-binder.

2. BANDAGING THE GROIN AND UPPER THIGH (*Spica of the Groin*) (three-inch bandage)

The groin and upper thigh are bandaged with a series of figure-of-eight turns around the lower abdomen and upper thigh. These turns may either ascend or descend.

147

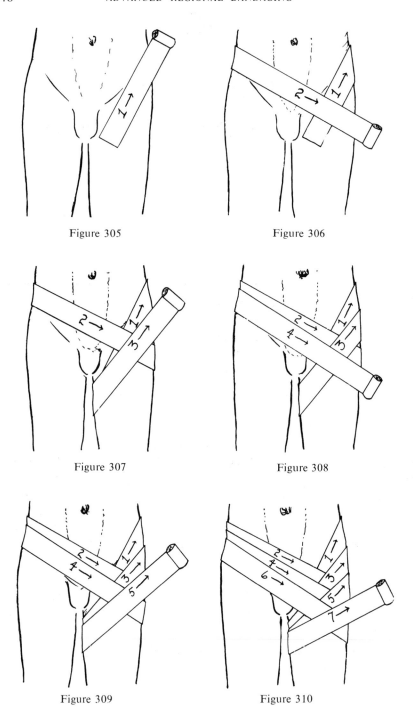

Figure 305

Figure 306

Figure 307

Figure 308

Figure 309

Figure 310

Directions

A. Anchor the bandage with an oblique turn which begins at the upper medial aspect of the thigh. Carry the roller obliquely upward and laterally over the groin. (See Fig. 305.) Encircle the lower abdomen and return to the thigh, crossing the initial extremity at an oblique angle. (See Fig. 306.) This completes the first loop of the figure-of-eight, and also serves to fix the bandage.

B. Apply an oblique turn around the upper thigh. (See Fig. 307.) This completes the second loop of the figure-of-eight.

C. Apply a second figure-of-eight turn, lower than, and partly overlapping, the first turn. (See Figs. 308, 309.)

D. Apply as many additional figure-of-eight turns as are necessary to completely cover the part. (See Fig. 310.)

3. BANDAGING BOTH GROINS *(Double Spica of Groins)* (three-inch bandage)

Both groins may be bandaged by applying alternating figure-of-eight turns to first one groin, and the abdomen, and then the other groin and the abdomen.

Directions

A. Proceed as though bandaging one groin. (See Figs. 305, 306, 307.)

B. After encircling the abdomen, instead of returning to the same thigh, carry the bandage obliquely downward over the opposite thigh and encircle same. (See Fig. 311.)

C. Carry the roller around the abdomen and return to the first thigh. (See Fig. 312.)

D. Repeat with these alternating figure-of-eight turns until both groins are covered.

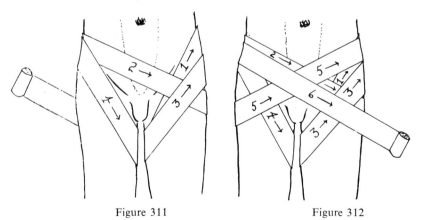

Figure 311   Figure 312

4. BANDAGING THE BUTTOCKS AND LATERAL THIGH (*Spica of Buttocks*) (three-inch bandage)

The upper lateral aspect of the thighs and the buttocks may be bandaged with a series of figure-of-eight turns, with loops around the thigh and abdomen. The point of crossing of the figure-of-eight turns can be so situated and placed as to cover the site of the injured area. (See Figs. 313, 314.)

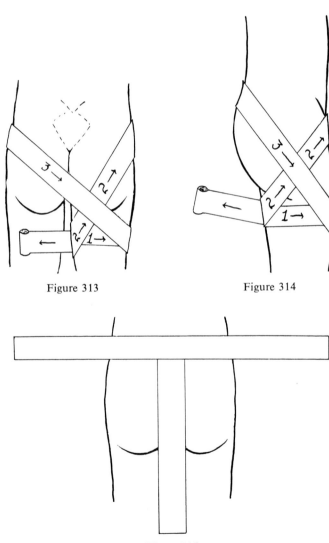

Figure 313   Figure 314

Figure 315

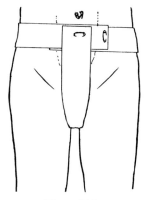

Figure 316

5. BANDAGING THE PERINEUM (*T-binder*)

The perineum can be bandaged with a series of figure-of-eight turns around both thighs, with the point of crossing over the perineum; however, this does not afford adequate pressure to the part. The best form of bandage for the perineum is the T-binder, with either the single-T, or double-T. The main part of the bandage is passed around the back, sides, and front of the abdomen and pinned there. The tail is carried under and around the perineum and is pinned to the transverse band anteriorly. (See Figs. 315, 316.)

UNIT FOUR ...

THE TRIANGULAR BANDAGE

CONTENTS OF UNIT FOUR

The Triangular Bandage

Chapter 21

Preparation of the Triangle

Chapter 22

Basic Principles and Technique of Use

Chapter 23

Regional Bandaging with the Triangle

21

Preparation of the Triangle

1. Introduction.
2. Preparation of the triangle.
3. Parts of the triangle.
4. The cravat bandage.

INTRODUCTION

The triangular bandage is a bandage made with a triangular-shaped piece of material. This bandage has found particular favor in first aid and emergency work for the temporary dressing of wounds, fractures, and dislocations because:

1. It is readily improvised from any kind of cloth, silk, shirt, sheet, pillowcase, handkerchief, or any other such material.
2. It is adaptable to any region of the body.
3. It is fairly easy to apply once the new fundamental principles of application have been mastered.
4. Properly applied, it serves its function well.

In fractures and other injuries not involving the skin, the triangle may be used alone. It must be remembered, however, that on open wounds, sterile dressings are first applied, the triangle serving merely to hold the dressings in place and support the parts.

PREPARATION OF THE TRIANGLE

The triangle is usually prepared from a square piece of material which is folded diagonally and then cut along the fold. This gives two triangles. If a square piece of material is not available, then a triangular-shaped piece of material may be cut directly. The size of the square used will vary with the circumstances and availability of material; however, whenever possible the material should be a 36–40 inch square before folding and cutting. For general hospital, Army, Navy, and Civilian Defense emergency work a supply of these triangles is prepared in advance and kept available for use. These are most commonly prepared from firm muslin. Ready-prepared triangles may be obtained from most of the commercial surgical supply houses.

PARTS OF THE TRIANGLE

The triangular bandage consists of: (See Fig. 317.)

1. *The Apex or Point:* The right angle of the triangle.
2. *The Base:* The longest side of the triangle, opposite the apex.
3. *The Ends or Extremities:* The acute angles.

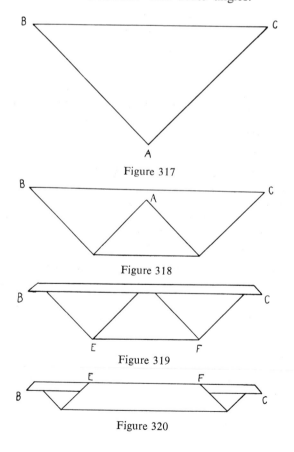

Figure 317

Figure 318

Figure 319

Figure 320

THE CRAVAT BANDAGE

In using the triangular bandage, it is often necessary to fold the triangle. This is done as follows:

Bring point A to within one inch of the midpoint or center of line BC. (See Fig. 318.) Fold the base (BC) back so as to cover point A. (See Fig. 319.) If this is too wide for use, it can be folded further. (See Fig. 320.) The triangle which has been folded several times in this way is referred to as the *Cravat Bandage.*

Both triangle and cravat bandages are sometimes referred to as the *Handkerchief Bandages,* since both were originally devised from a large handkerchief by M. Mayor, a Swiss surgeon.

22

Basic Principles and Technique of Use

---

1. The functional approach.
2. Methods of fixation.
3. The reef or square knot.
4. Naming of triangle bandages.
5. Axioms for good application.

---

1. THE FUNCTIONAL APPROACH

The functional bandager, aiming for efficiency, speed, and neatness, will realize that there are several simple principles involved in the application of the triangle and cravat bandages. Having familiarized himself with these fundamental ideas, he finds little difficulty in applying these bandages to any part of the body.

There is a central *application site* or *useful area* of the triangle or cravat which is applied to the injured area or over a dressing. (See Figs. 321, 322.) The ends and the apex are then used merely to tie the bandage in place and fix the injured part in the desired position. This is the entire working principle of application of the triangle.

In the application of the cravat, several additional points must be kept in mind. The center of the cravat is applied over the dressing on the injured area. First one end (*B* or *C*) is carried around the injured part. Then the second end (*C* or *B*) is carried around in the opposite direction; thus, one end at a time completes its turn. Finally, the two ends are tied. These principles are best illustrated in the following chapter in which the cravat is used for holding a dressing in place over the palm of the hand.

158

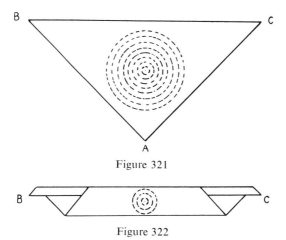

Figure 321

Figure 322

2. METHODS OF FIXATION

The triangle, or cravat, is fixed and held in place either by tying the ends, or by pinning it in place with safety pins. To facilitate knot tying with the ends of the triangle, the base is folded upon itself for a distance of one inch, as described previously. (See Fig. 319, in folding the triangle.) In tying the ends of the triangle, or cravat, it is recommended that the *reef* or *square knot* be used in preference to the granny knot, since it is less likely to slip than the latter.

3. THE REEF OR SQUARE KNOT

With one end of the triangle in each hand, the knot is prepared as follows:

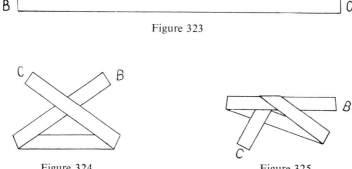

B ——————————————————— C

Figure 323

Figure 324   Figure 325

The right end (*C*) is passed over, around, and under the left end (*B*). (See Figs. 323, 324, 325.) The hands are changed and the first half of the knot completed by pulling the ends. The left end (*C*) is now passed over, around, and under the right end (*B*). (See Figs. 326, 327.) The hands are then changed and the second half of the knot completed by pulling the ends. This gives the reef or square knot, which does not slip. When the knot is completed, the ends should be neatly tucked beneath the bandage.

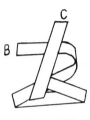

Figure 326

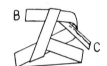

Figure 327

4. NAMING OF TRIANGLE BANDAGES

It is interesting to note that in the past a wide variety of names was used to designate the various applications of the triangle. Thus, from the title of the bandage, the bandager could determine the mode of application. The first part of the title indicated the region to which the *base* was applied; the second part indicated the region over which the *ends* were tied. For example, the *occipito-frontal triangle* was applied with the base over the occiput and the apex and the ends tied over the frontal region.

Having learned the basic principles of application of the triangle, the bandager need not be concerned with the titles these bear, especially since most of these names are now obsolete.

5. AXIOMS FOR GOOD APPLICATION

1. The knot should be placed in such a position that it does not cause discomfort or pain to any part. It should not be placed over pressure points, such as the back of the neck, the axilla, the back, and the buttocks.
2. When a triangle passes tightly under the axilla or over the perineum, a pad should first be applied, so as to protect the delicate skin surfaces.
3. No portion of the triangle should be allowed to hang loosely. All parts should be taut and firmly applied.

23

Regional Bandaging with the Triangle

1. Slings for the hand, forearm, and the arm.
2. Triangle for the scalp.
3. Triangle for the temple, forehead, and chin.
4. Triangle for fractured clavicle.
5. Triangle for the shoulder.
6. Triangle for the scapula.
7. Triangle for the upper arm.
8. Triangle for the hand.
9. Triangle for the chest.
10. Triangle for the hip and thigh.
11. Triangle for the knee.
12. Triangle for the foot.
13. Triangle for an amputation stump.
14. Triangle for the palm of the hand (the cravat bandage).

1. SLINGS FOR THE HAND, FOREARM, AND THE ARM

Uses: In injuries of the fingers, hand, wrist, forearm, and arm, it is usually desirable to rest the part and elevate it above its normal position. The sling is used for this support. In injuries of the shoulder and clavicle, the sling supports the arm, elbow, and forearm, thereby lessening the strain on, and pain in, the injured part. Not only do slings support the parts, but, properly applied, they may partly serve as immobilization dressings as well.

Types of Slings: There are various types of slings, depending on the particular indications for same. These are:

161

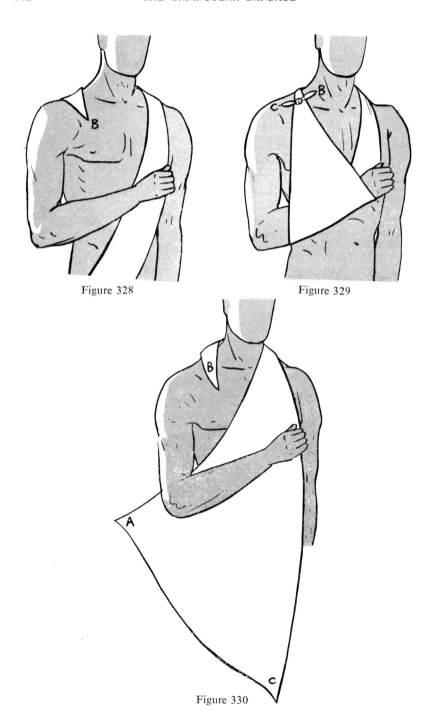

Figure 328

Figure 329

Figure 330

1. *Narrow Sling:* This is used for injuries of the fingers, hand, or wrist, and is prepared as follows:

(a) Fold the triangle into a wide cravat.

(b) Place one end of the cravat (*B*) over the shoulder of the sound side, across the back of the neck on to the shoulder of the injured side. (See Fig. 328.)

(c) Place the injured hand across the body, above the level of the waist. (See Fig. 328.)

(d) Bring the other end (*C*) up and tie it to end (*B*). (See Fig. 329.)

2. *Broad Sling* (low): This type of sling is the most commonly used and most comfortable, since it lends support to the arms, elbow, forearm, wrist, and hand. It is prepared as follows:

(a) Bring the apex (*A*) well under the arm of the injured side, and place one of the ends (*B*) over the opposite shoulder and around the neck. (See Fig. 330.)

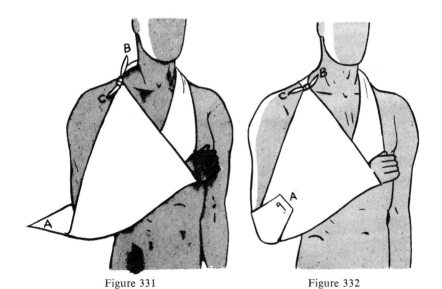

Figure 331   Figure 332

(b) Bring the arm across the chest, above the level of the waist. (See Fig. 330.)

(c) Bring up the other end (*C*) and tie it to end *B* over the shoulder on the side of the injury. (See Fig. 331.) It is important in this step to bring end *C* high enough, otherwise the sling will not afford adequate support. Include the hand in the sling.

(d) Fold the apex (*A*) over the elbow and pin it in place. (See Fig. 332.)

3. *Broad Sling* (high): This type of sling may be used instead of the low sling; however, it has the added advantage that the forearm can be more readily adjusted to any desired height. It is particularly valuable in fractures of the clavicle. It is prepared as follows:

(a) Apply the base of the triangle (*BC*) to the injured side, with one end (*B*) over the shoulder, around the neck, and over the sound shoulder. (See Fig. 333.)

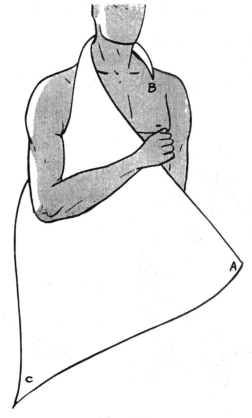

Figure 333

(b) Elevate the hand of the injured side so that it rests in front of the opposite shoulder. (See Fig. 333.)

(c) Bring the other end (*C*) up, and tie it to end *B* over the sound shoulder. (See Fig. 334.)

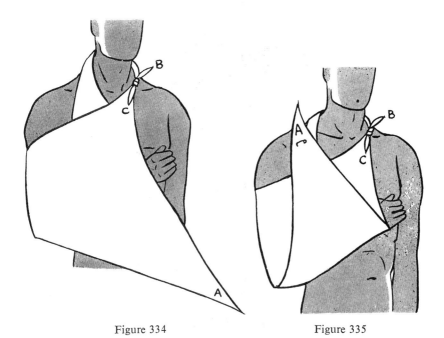

Figure 334   Figure 335

(d) Bring the apex (*A*) up and pin it on the shoulder of the injured side. (See Fig. 335.) The height of the elevated forearm can be controlled by the height to which the apex is elevated. A pad should be placed in the axilla of the injured side.

2. TRIANGLE FOR THE SCALP

This bandage covers the entire scalp and thus may be used for covering dressings over any and all parts of the scalp. It is prepared as follows:

(a) Apply the middle of the base (*BC*) to the forehead, just above the level of the eyebrows, with the apex (*A*) hanging down over the back of the head. (See Fig. 336.)

(b) Carry the two ends (*B* and *C*) backward, above the ears, and cross them over the back of the head. (See Fig. 337.)

(c) Carry the ends to the front of the head and tie over the forehead. (See Figs. 338, 339.)

(d) Pull the apex (*A*) downward so that it fits tightly to the scalp, and then carry it on to the top of the head. Pin it in place here. (See Fig. 340.)

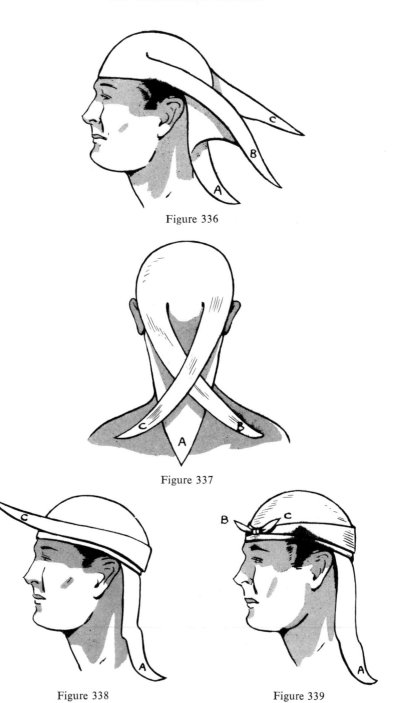

Figure 336

Figure 337

Figure 338

Figure 339

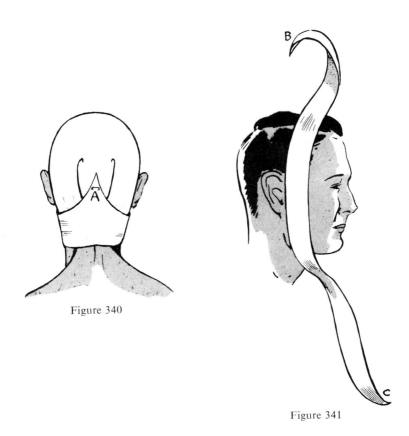

Figure 340

Figure 341

3. TRIANGLE FOR THE TEMPLE, FOREHEAD, OR CHIN

This bandage is applicable for holding dressings in place over the forehead, the temple, or the lower jaw. It is applied as follows:

(a) Fold a triangle to a narrow cravat.

(b) Place the center of the cravat over the uninjured temple. (See Fig. 341.)

(c) Carry one end of the bandage (B or C) over the top of the head and the other end (C or B) under the jaw. (See Fig. 342.)

(d) Cross the ends around each other, over the dressing on the wound. (See Fig. 343.)

(e) Continue one end around the front of the head and the other around the back. (See Fig. 344.)

(f) Tie the ends on the uninjured side. (See Fig. 345.)

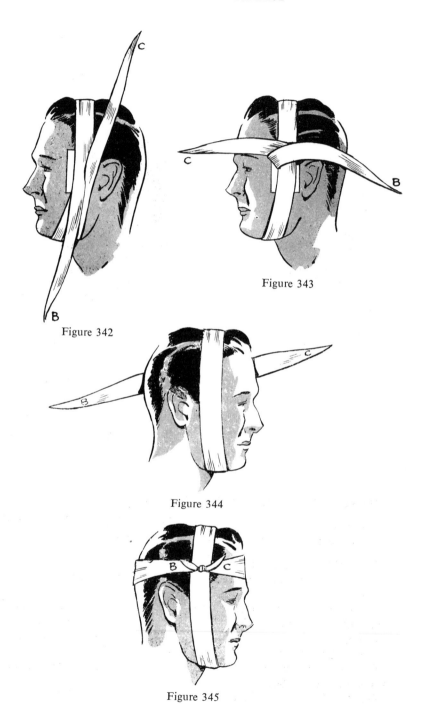

Figure 342

Figure 343

Figure 344

Figure 345

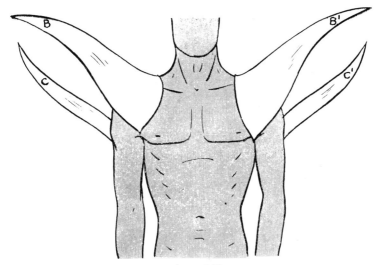

Figure 346

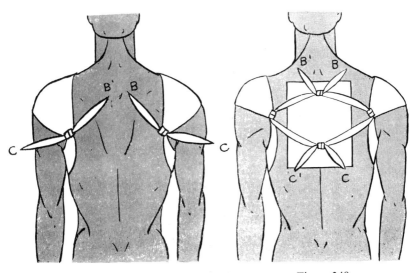

Figure 347   Figure 348

4. TRIANGLE FOR FRACTURED CLAVICLES (*collarbones*)

In fractures of the clavicles, the object of bandaging is to draw the shoulders back. This is done as follows:

(a) Fold two triangles to narrow cravats and apply to the shoulders as illustrated. (See Fig. 346.)

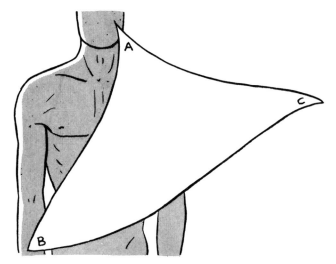

Figure 349

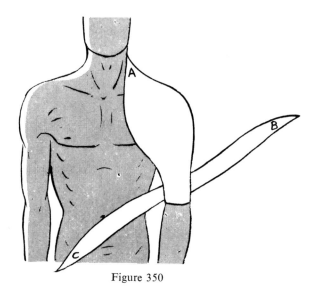

Figure 350

(b) Tie the cravats over the backs of the shoulders. (See Fig. 347.)

(c) Tie the upper strands of the cravats firmly together across the upper back; tie the lower strands in a similar fashion. (See Fig. 348.) Place a thick pad beneath the knots. (See Fig. 348.) The thicker the pad, the more effective the bandage.

(d) Support both the hands in a narrow sling.

5. TRIANGLE FOR THE SHOULDER

This bandage may be used for a variety of injuries to the shoulder and upper arm. It is prepared as follows:

(a) Apply the base (*BC*) of the triangle to the arm, allowing the apex (*A*) to rest on the shoulder. (See Fig. 349.)

(b) Cross the ends (*B* and *C*) behind the arm. (See Fig. 350.)

(c) Tie the ends (*B* and *C*) around the front of the arm. (See Fig. 351.)

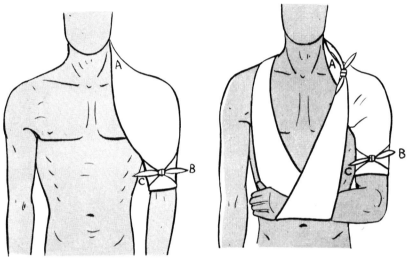

Figure 351   Figure 352

(d) Elevate the forearm of the injured side in a narrow sling, catching the apex (*A*) of the triangle under the sling. (See Fig. 352.)

(e) Fold the apex (*A*) down over the knot of the sling, and pin it to the bandage on the shoulder. (See Fig. 353.)

(f) If the injury is of such a nature that the arm cannot be supported in a sling, then a narrow cravat is used. Place the center of the cravat over the apex (*A*) of the shoulder bandage, carry the ends of the cravat across the front and back of the chest, and tie the ends in front of the axilla of the uninjured side. Pin the apex (*A*) of the shoulder bandage over the cravat. (See Fig. 354.)

6. TRIANGLE FOR THE SCAPULA (*shoulder blade*)

The purpose of this dressing is to immobilize the fractured bone, and therefore it must be firmly applied. The bandage is prepared as follows:

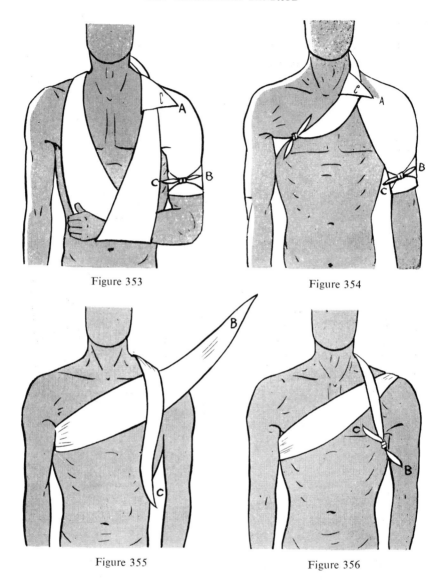

Figure 353

Figure 354

Figure 355

Figure 356

(a) Apply a soft pad to each axilla.

(b) Fold a triangle so as to form a wide cravat.

(c) Place the center of the cravat under the axilla of the injured side and carry the ends (B and C) around the chest and over the shoulder of the uninjured side. (See Fig. 355.)

(d) Cross the ends (B and C) over the shoulder and tie in front of the axilla of the uninjured side. (See Fig. 356.)

(e) Support the arm of the injured side in a sling.

7. TRIANGLE FOR THE UPPER ARM

This dressing immobilizes the upper arm and compresses it firmly against the chest wall. It is of value in fractures of the humerus. It is applied as follows:

(a) Fold a triangle to a wide cravat, and apply the center to the upper part of the injured arm.

(b) Carry the ends (*B* and *C*) around the chest and tie in front of the opposite axilla. (See Fig. 357.)

(c) Support the wrist of the injured arm in a narrow sling. (See Fig. 358.)

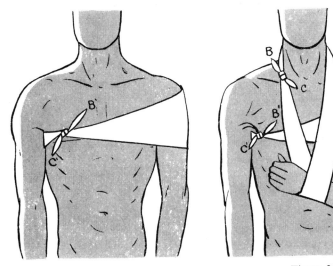

Figure 357   Figure 358

8. TRIANGLE FOR THE HAND

This bandage is applicable to wounds of the fingers, palm, or dorsum of the hand. It is readily applied as follows:

(a) Place the hand on the triangle so that the base (*BC*) lies at the level of the wrist. (See Fig. 359.)

(b) Turn the apex (*A*) over the hand as far as it will go. Properly applied, the apex (*A*) will extend slightly higher up on the wrist than the base (*BC*). This allows for more efficient tying later. (See Fig. 360.)

(c) Turn the sides of the triangle in. (See Fig. 361.)

(d) Carry the ends around the wrist, leaving the apex (*A*) exposed. (See Fig. 362.)

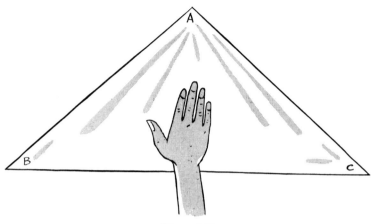

Figure 359

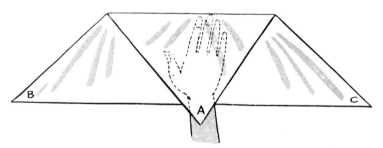

Figure 360

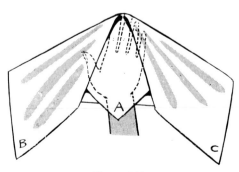

Figure 361

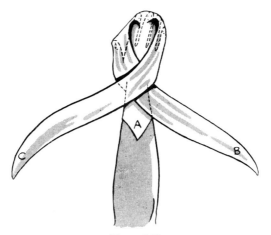

Figure 362

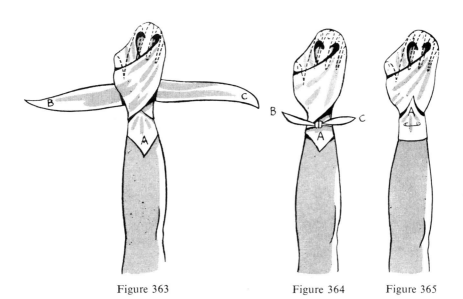

Figure 363   Figure 364   Figure 365

(e) Cross the ends (*B* and *C*) in front of the wrist. (See Fig. 363.)

(f) Tie the ends (*B* and *C*) on the back of the wrist. (See Fig. 364.)

(g) Carry the apex (*A*) down over the knot and pin it to the bandage. (See Fig. 365.)

9. TRIANGLE FOR THE CHEST

This bandage may be used very effectively in covering wide areas of the chest. It is applied as follows:

(a) Place the base (*BC*) of the triangle across the chest with the apex (*A*) over the shoulder of the injured side. (See Fig. 366.)

(b) Carry the two ends (*B* and *C*) around the chest to the back. (See Fig. 367.)

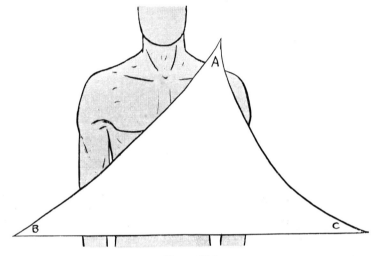

Figure 366

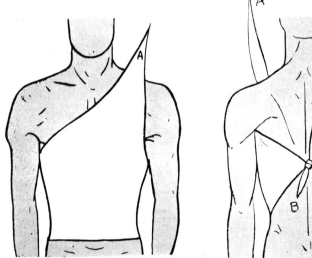

Figure 367

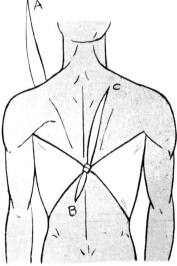

Figure 368

(c) Tie the ends (*B* and *C*) so that one is longer than the other. (See Fig. 368.)

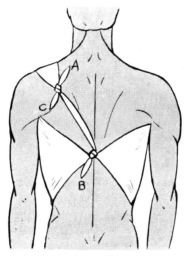

Figure 369

(d) Carry the longer end to the shoulder and tie it to the apex (*A*). (See Fig. 369.)

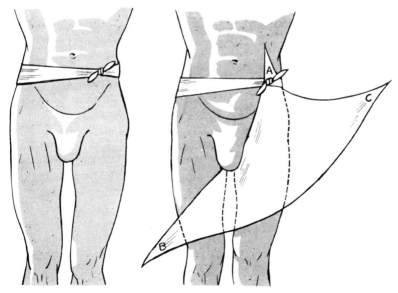

Figure 370   Figure 371

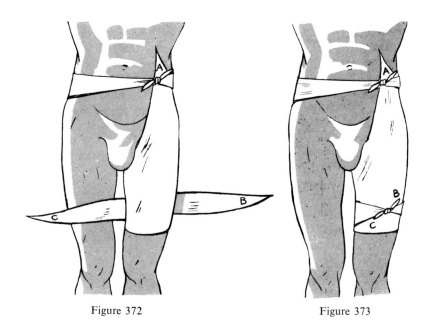

Figure 372   Figure 373

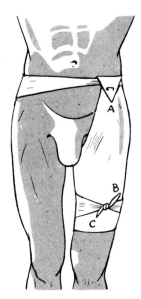

Figure 374

10. TRIANGLE FOR THE HIP AND THIGH

This bandage may be used for covering the upper thigh, the hip, and the gluteal regions. It is applied as follows:

(a) Fold a triangle to a narrow cravat, and tie around the waist, with the knot on the side of the injured thigh or hip. (See Fig. 370.)

(b) Apply a triangle to the hip so that the apex (A) slides under the cravat and the base (BC) is applied to the thigh. (See Fig. 371.)

(c) Carry the two ends (B and C) around the thigh and tie. (See Figs. 372, 373.)

(d) Fold the apex (A) down over the knot in the cravat, and pin it in place. (See Fig. 374.)

11. TRIANGLE FOR THE KNEE

In applying the knee bandage, the knee should be kept in a partly flexed position. The bandage is applied as follows:

(a) Place the center of the base (BC) just below the kneecap, with the apex (A) up on the thigh. (See Fig. 375.)

(b) Carry the ends (B and C) around and cross them behind the knee. (See Fig. 376.)

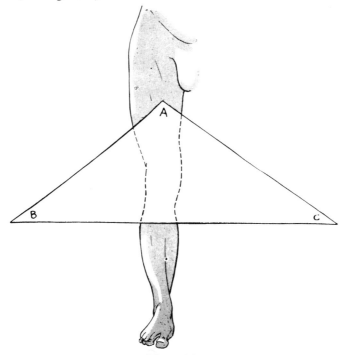

Figure 375

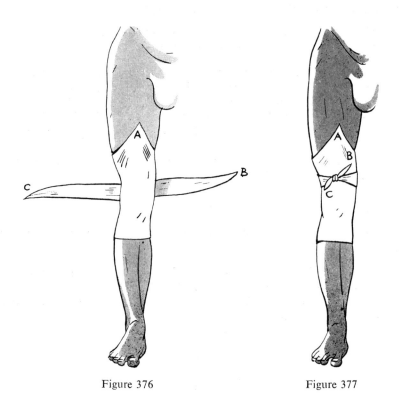

Figure 376   Figure 377

(c) Bring the ends (*B* and *C*) forward and tie them above the knee. (See Fig. 377.)

(d) Pull the apex (*A*) down over the knot and pin it in place. (See Fig. 378.)

12. TRIANGLE FOR THE FOOT

This dressing is valuable for bandaging the toes, the foot, the heel, and the ankle. Its application is similar to that of the triangle of the hand. It is prepared as follows:

(a) Place the foot upon the center of a triangle, with the toes pointing toward the apex (*A*), and the heel of the foot about four inches from the base (*BC*). (See Fig. 379.)

(b) Bring the apex (*A*) up over the foot. (See Fig. 380.)

(c) Pick up the ends (*B* and *C*) and carry them across the front of the foot. Bring first one across and then the other. (See Figs. 381, 382.)

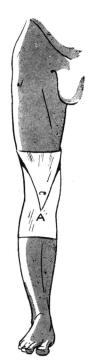

Figure 378

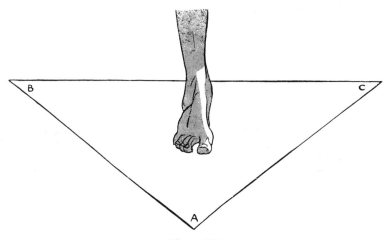

Figure 379

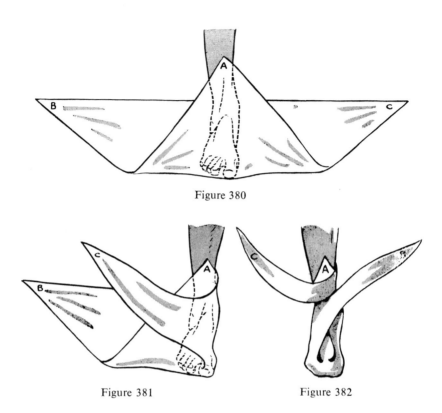

Figure 380

Figure 381   Figure 382

(d) Carry the ends around the back of the foot. (See Fig. 383.)
(e) Tie the ends (*B* and *C*) over the front of the foot. (See Fig. 384.)

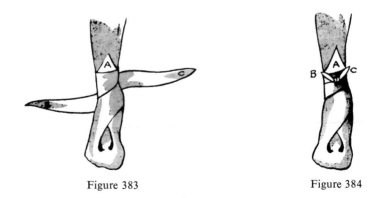

Figure 383   Figure 384

(f) Fold the apex (*A*) down over the knot and pin it in place. (See Fig. 385.)

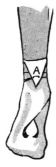

Figure 385

13. TRIANGLE FOR AN AMPUTATION STUMP

This is somewhat similar to the hand bandage, described earlier in this chapter. It is applied as follows:

(a) Place the base (*BC*) against the posterior aspect of the stump, with the apex (*A*) hanging down. (See Fig. 386.)

(b) Carry the apex (*A*) over the stump. (See Fig. 387.)

(c) Carry the ends around the stump, one crossing the other. (See Figs. 388, 389.)

(d) Bring the ends (*B* and *C*) around to the front and tie. (See Fig. 390.)

(e) Fold the apex (*A*) down over the knot and pin it in place. (See Fig. 391.)

14. CRAVAT FOR PALM OF THE HAND

Although the following bandage is used for the palm, it demonstrates the basic principles involved in the application of the cravat: namely, that one end at a time completes its turn before the other end is carried around the part. In this manner a neat, well applied dressing is produced. The basic principles illustrated here are applicable in the preparation of cravat bandages for the neck, forearm, arm, wrist, thigh, and leg.

(a) Fold the triangle to a narrow cravat.

(b) Apply the center of the cravat over the dressing on the palm. (See Fig. 392.)

(c) Carry one end (*C*) around the back of the hand. (See Fig. 393.)

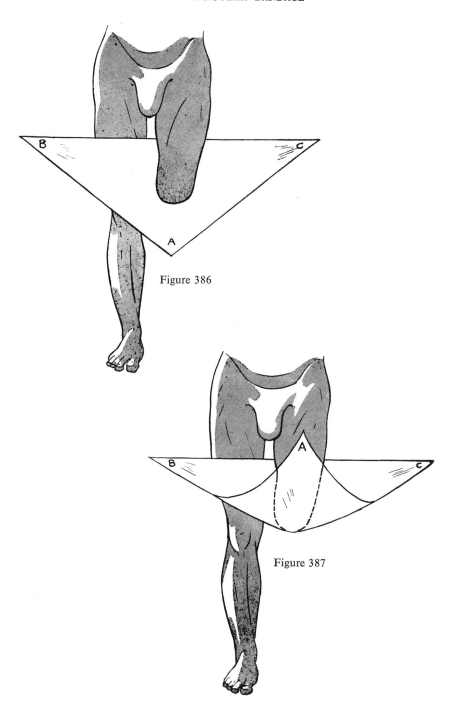

Figure 386

Figure 387

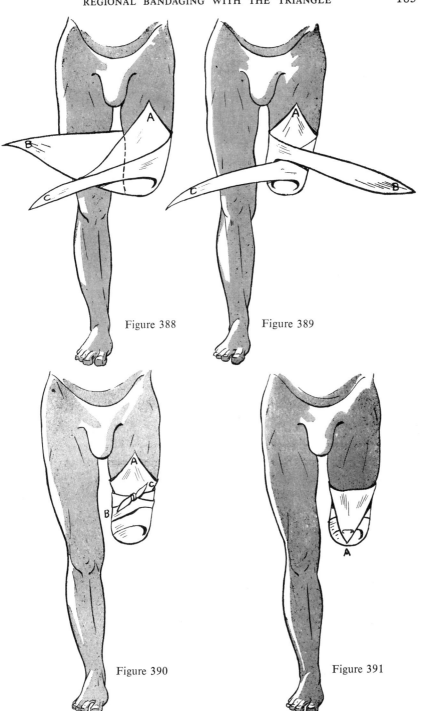

Figure 388

Figure 389

Figure 390

Figure 391

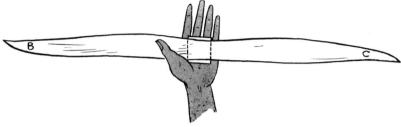

Figure 392

(d) Carry the second end (B) around the back of the hand in the opposite direction. (See Fig. 394.) A posterior view of the ends as they cross over the back of the hand is illustrated. (See Fig. 395.)

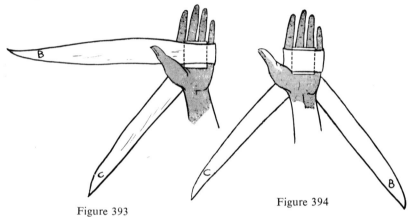

Figure 393

Figure 394

(e) Carry the ends (B and C), one at a time, around to the front of the wrist. (See Fig. 396.)

(f) Tie the ends behind the wrist. (See Fig. 397.)

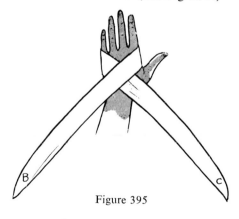

Figure 395

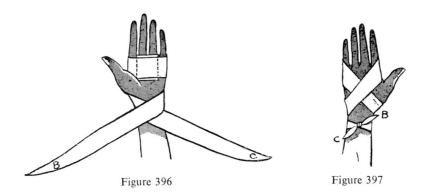

Figure 396   Figure 397

Note that in the above-described dressing, the cravat has really formed a figure-of-eight bandage around the hand and the wrist. In bandaging the cylinder and cone-shaped parts, such as the forearm, arm, thigh, and leg, first one end is carried around the part, and then the other is carried around in the oppositite direction, until finally the ends are short enough to tie.

UNIT FIVE ...

TAPING AND ADHESIVE PLASTER DRESSINGS

24

Adhesive Plaster Dressings and Taping

1. Introduction.
2. Uses of adhesive plaster in surgery.
3. Types of adhesive plaster:
   (a) Regular type.
   (b) Waterproof adhesive plaster.
   (c) Special strapping plaster.
4. Principles of application and preparation of skin surfaces.
5. Practical applications:
   (a) Starting and terminating of bandages.
   (b) Fixation of surgical dressings.
   (c) Adhesive as a substitute for suture in small wounds.
   (d) Adhesive in large, unsutured wounds.
   (e) Adhesive plaster immobilization—"taping."
   (f) Skin traction in the treatment of fractures.
   (g) Adhesive plaster in bivalved casts.
   (h) Adhesive plaster in epithelialization of wounds.
6. Removal of adhesive plaster.

1. INTRODUCTION

As its name implies, adhesive plaster is a form of bandaging material used for its ability to adhere firmly to surfaces. The uses of adhesive plaster are innumerable, and outside the field of surgery this material has found extensive application almost equal in scope to its use in surgery. These include the temporary repair of cracked glass windows, automobile canvas tops, and book covers, the covering of tennis racquet and golf club handles, and other uses too numerous to mention.

191

2. USES OF ADHESIVE PLASTER IN SURGERY

In surgery, adhesive plaster has found a similarly diversified field of application. The main uses are:

(a) To fix bandages;
(b) to hold dressings in place;
(c) to replace sutures in the repair of small wounds;
(d) to aid in the approximation of skin surfaces in large gaping wounds which are not sutured;
(e) to immobilize and support various parts of the body;
(f) to maintain traction in the treatment of fractures;
(g) to hold bivalved casts in place;
(h) to encourage epithelialization in wounds.

Each of these uses will be elaborated upon later in this chapter.

3. TYPES OF ADHESIVE PLASTER

Adhesive plaster is prepared by spreading a mixture of zinc oxide, waxes, resin, and rubber onto one surface of a firm, closely woven cotton material. The material is cut to various widths and then wound on spools in which form it is ready for use. The spools of adhesive vary from ¼ inch up to 12 inches in width, and from one yard up to 10 yards in length. (See Fig. 398.)

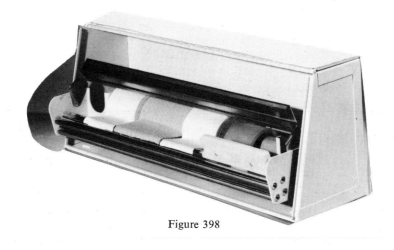

Figure 398

There are three basic types of adhesive plaster. These include:
Regular Type: This is the most commonly used form of adhesive plaster and is prepared as described above.

Waterproof Adhesive Plaster: This is similar to the regular type except that the back cloth is specially coated with a waterproof substance. This type of plaster is preferable for dressings which require protection from wetting and soiling.

Special Strapping Adhesive Plasters: These plasters are prepared specially for use in traumatic and orthopedic surgery where great tensile strength is required. Instead of the ordinary cotton material, strong moleskin and other specially woven materials are employed as back cloths.

4. PRINCIPLES OF APPLICATION AND PREPARATION OF SKIN SURFACES

Adhesive plaster should be applied to clean surfaces. Small traces of oil, grease, glycerine, and similar substances interfere with adhesion. The same is true of moist surfaces, or surfaces covered with a film of dust, or powder. The skin must be reasonably clean and dry.

Adequate preparation of the skin includes, first, the shaving of the part if there is a moderate or more than moderate amount of hair. The skin is thoroughly cleansed with liberal amounts of soap and water and then dried. Either alcohol or ether is then applied to remove any fatty material that may have remained and also to aid further in the drying of the part.

When adhesive plaster is applied to a surface for any length of time, certain factors are introduced which merit consideration:

   a. Retention of sweat and oily secretions of the skin, with resultant softening of the skin;
   b. Maceration of the skin by friction; and
   c. Trauma to skin capillaries.

In addition to these skin changes, certain persons have shown various reactions to adhesive plaster, characterized by redness, swelling, and even blistering of the skin. These have been attributed to some special sensitivity to any or all of the ingredients in the adherent mass on the plaster. For this reason, various modifications have been made in the adherent material to produce a minimum of skin reaction.

Furthermore, some products have been produced which are highly porous, allowing for escape of perspiration and skin exudates through the adhesive plaster. Micropore® and Dermicel® tape, in addition to being highly porous, have the added advantage of easy removal from hairy surfaces without pulling out the hair. Furthermore, these remain adherent even on immersion into water.

In spite of these much-improved products, some skins are so delicate as to react to any of these, or possibly just to the trauma of being taped.

This trauma to the skin can be minimized by an additional step in the preparation of same. Following the preliminary washing and drying, the skin is covered with a liquid substance which, when dry, forms a protective coating over the skin, to which the adhesive is then applied. Numerous materials have been used for this purpose. These include:

Tincture of Benzoin: This is a brown resinous substance which is applied by means of a cotton applicator. When dry it forms a thin, sticky film which protects the skin and aids in adhesion of the plaster to the skin.

Mercurochrome: A one per cent aqueous solution of mercurochrome is applied by means of a swab, or cotton applicator. After it is dry, a second and even third coat may be applied.

Collodion: Collodion, a solution of guncotton in ether and alcohol, when applied and allowed to dry, forms a thin, transparent, flexible coating. It has an added advantage over the previously described substances in that, if applied in sufficient quantity and thickness, it eliminates the necessity for shaving off the hair. In drying it incorporates the hair in the film and thus the hair is not pulled upon when the adhesive is removed.

Special Commercial Products: Various commercial products have been recommended for the purpose of protecting the skin from adhesives and for maintaining greater adhesion of the plaster with less slipping. Ace Adherent® is a colorless solution which dries to an extremely sticky surface, ideal for the prevention of slipping of the adhesive tape. Aeroplast® is a plastic which is sprayed onto the surface, forming a protective film coating for the skin. Benzoin may also be dispensed through a spray can.

Often considerable difficulty is encountered in making adhesive plaster stick to the skin. Slight heating of the sticky surface over a match or alcohol flame will usually remedy this difficulty. Moistening the sticky surface of the adhesive with a small amount of alcohol, or ether, just prior to application, will aid in better fixation of the plaster to the skin surface.

Large strappings made with waterproof adhesive plaster may come loose on patients who perspire freely. The waterproof backing interferes with evaporation, causing the moisture to accumulate under the plaster and loosen it. In these cases, the regular adhesive plaster, or highly porous plaster, is recommended. It is interesting to note that the punctate mottling of adhesive plaster, often seen after prolonged application, is produced by the oily secretions from the sebaceous glands of the skin.

5. PRACTICAL APPLICATIONS

Starting and Terminating of Bandages

In the application of the roller bandage, adhesive plaster finds two main uses:

(a) *Starting the Bandage:* Adhesive plaster serves to anchor the initial extremity of the roller. A strip of adhesive, about 1 inch wide and 3 to 4 inches long, is applied, with one-half on the bandage and one-half on the skin surface. (See Fig. 399.)

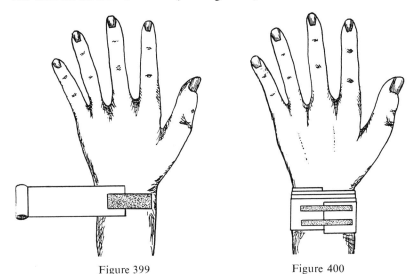

Figure 399   Figure 400

(b) *Terminating the Bandage:* Most commonly, a small strip of adhesive plaster, 3 to 4 inches long and ½ to 1 inch wide, is applied partly to the final turn of a bandage and partly to the underlying previous turn. (See Fig. 89.) It is recommended that in preference to this method, two narrow strips, each about ½ inch wide, be applied, as illustrated. (See Fig. 400.) This makes for firmer support.

Fixation of Surgical Dressings

The fixation and maintenance in place of surgical dressings is one of the most important uses of adhesive plaster in surgery. Innumerable methods have been devised and employed for the most advantageous use in this respect. These vary from the very simple to rather complex methods. Following are some of the most commonly used methods of application:

(a) *Small Wounds:* These include small superficial wounds over most any part of the body. A sterile dressing is placed over the wound and one or more strips of adhesive are applied, depending upon the size of the wound. The application of a single strip of adhesive across the dressing is referred to as *line taping.* (See Fig. 401.) The application of two strips at right angles to each other is called *cross taping.* (See Fig. 402.) In Fig. 403, note that first a horizontal and then a vertical strip are applied. Then a second horizontal and a second vertical strip are applied respectively. This makes for a firmer, less readily loosened dressing than if first two

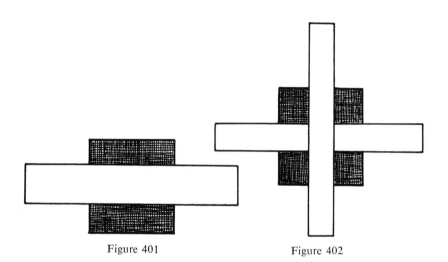

Figure 401   Figure 402

horizontal and then two vertical strips were applied. This method of application is referred to as *hatch taping.*

(b) *Large Wounds:* Following the repair of large or deep traumatic or operative wounds, sterile dressings are applied. Over the extremities these dressings are held in place by roller bandages, which may then be firmly fixed by adhesive plaster as described earlier. However, in chest and abdominal wounds, it is not very easy or practical to apply these roller bandages and thus adhesive plaster is used directly for holding the dressings in place. Long strips of adhesive, 12 to 15 inches long and 2 to 3 inches wide, are placed across the dressing, the number of strips depending on the size of the dressing. (See Fig. 404.)

It may be desirable, and often necessary, to examine the wounds from time to time, and thus removal of the adhesive at each examination exposes the skin to considerable unnecessary trauma and irritation. This is particularly the case in infected and draining wounds which may require as many as three to four daily changes. For this reason various means have been devised to obviate the necessity for complete removal of the adhesive each time. A more or less "temporarily permanent" ad-

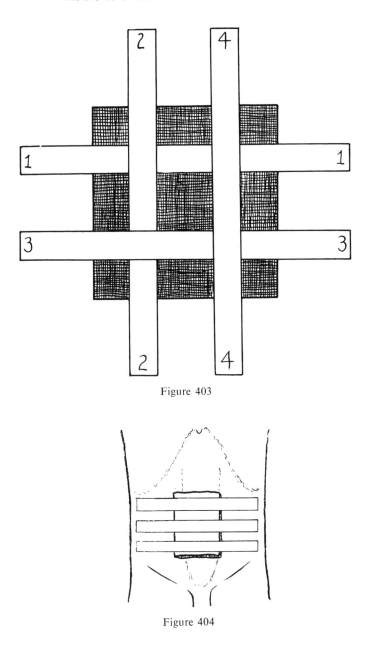

Figure 403

Figure 404

hesive device is used. Although various names have been applied to this method such as *Montgomery tapes,* adhesive straps, ties, corsets, and binders, the basic principles are the same.

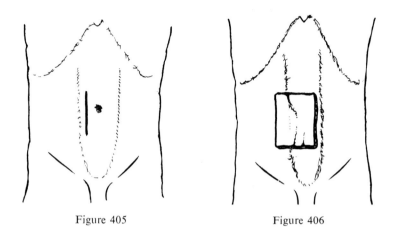

Figure 405   Figure 406

Following is the fundamental preparation: Assume that an abdominal wound, 5 inches long, is to be dressed. (See Fig. 405.)

The sterile dressings are applied. (See Fig. 406.)

Two strips of adhesive plaster, each about 12 inches long and 7 inches wide, are prepared. (See Fig. 407.)

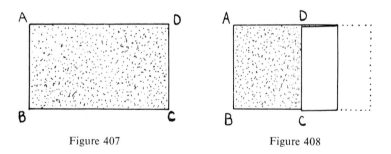

Figure 407   Figure 408

Each strip is folded back upon itself for a distance of 3 inches, bringing the two adherent surfaces together. (See Fig. 408.)

Several holes are made in the double-layered nonadherent portion at intervals of 1 inch apart, along a line about one-half inch from the free border. (See Fig. 409.) To reinforce the free border of the adhesive, a narrow piece of paper cardboard may be inserted and incorporated into the free border prior to the folding back of the strip. (See Fig. 410.) The holes are then made through the inserted material. Metal eyelets or hooks are placed in these holes to facilitate lacing of the parts. These make for a firmer border and one which may withstand greater tension and strain.

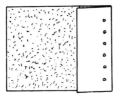

Figure 409

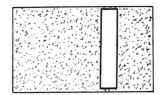

Figure 410

These are now ready for application and are applied to the body, one to the right and the other to the left of the wound dressing. These must be so applied that no portion of the adhesive part of the strip comes into contact with the dressing, the latter lying in contact with the non-adherent portion only. (See Fig. 411.)

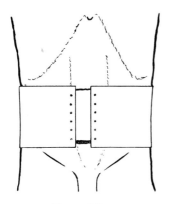

Figure 411

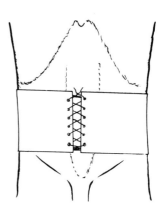

Figure 412

The adhesive portion is applied firmly to the skin on the lateral and posterior parts of the abdomen. The two adhesive strips are now tied with a string, lace, or gauze tape. (See Fig. 412.) With this method, to change a dressing, one has merely to untie the lace or string and fold back the nonadherent portion of the adhesive. These strips may be left in place until the wound is completely healed. Occasionally, in profusely draining wounds with spill over the adhesive tapes, complete removal and change of the adhesive may be necessary.

Instead of a wide strip of adhesive, several smaller strips may be prepared in a similar fashion and applied. (See Fig. 413.)

The wider strips are usually prepared in advance and stored, with application when necessary. The narrow strips are often applied after the original wider strips have been removed. If no cardboard is available, these narrow strips may be reinforced with tongue depressors which may

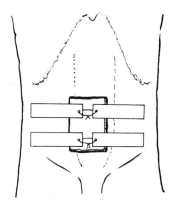

Figure 413

be cut or broken to the proper size. It is important, in using either the cardboard or tongue depressor reinforcement, that neither of these extends beyond the upper or lower border of the adhesive dressing, since these may serve as points of irritation and discomfort to the patient.

These so-called *Montgomery ties* may be obtained commercially, ready-prepared, in wide strips which may then be cut to any desired size. (See Fig. 414.)

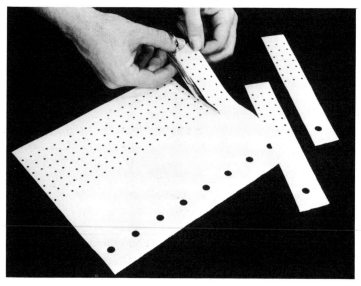

Figure 414

Adhesive Plaster as a Substitute for Suture in Small Wounds

In the closure of small lacerations of the skin, adhesive plaster may often satisfactorily be used instead of suture materials. In such wounds, particularly those on the scalp, face, and neck, the repair and healing is often as good as that which may be obtained with the use of suture material. Where needle and suture material are not available, adhesive certainly makes a reliable substitute.

The adhesive is applied in the form of a "butterfly" or "dumbbell," both of these terms being more or less descriptive of the shape of adhesive strip applied.

A piece of adhesive plaster is cut in such fashion as to have two wide portions connected by a narrow central bridge. (See Figs. 415, 416.) The adhesive is cut along the dotted line indicated in Fig. 415.

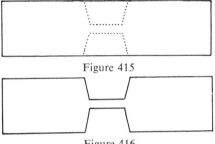

Figure 415

Figure 416

The purpose of this shape is to have only a small portion of the adhesive in contact with the wound, while a large surface of the material is in contact with the skin on each side of the wound, to give adequate traction. The narrow center allows for free drainage from the wound.

The application is as follows: With the ends of the strip supported in each hand, the narrow center is flamed over either a match or alcohol flame. The adhesive strip is first applied to the skin on one side of the wound. It is then drawn toward and applied to the other side of the wound, thereby approximating the skin edges. (See Figs. 417, 418.) A

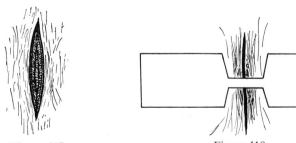

Figure 417

Figure 418

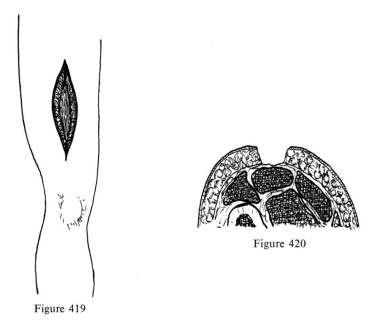

Figure 420

Figure 419

sterile dressing is then applied to the wound and held in place with adhesive strips.

Occasionally, even in those wounds in which one or two skin sutures have been inserted, *butterfly adhesives* are applied as additional aids to maintain adequate approximation of the skin surfaces. Adhesive *butterflies* are often applied to wounds which tend to gape slightly after the removal of sutures. In such wounds they keep the edges approximated until adequate healing has taken place. Sterile, ready-packaged strips of adhesive, ¼ by 3 inches, ready for adhesive closure of wounds, are available under the name of Steri-Strip®.

Adhesive Plaster in Large, Unsutured Wounds

The closure and approximation of skin surfaces in large, unsutured wounds is usually a long, drawn-out process, taxing the patience of even the most fastidious and careful surgical dresser. Following incision and drainage of large abscesses in the thigh or leg, or even in the abdominal wall, or following wide and extensive débridement of large traumatic wounds which are seen too late for tight suture closure, there is usually a very prolonged period of healing of the skin. This is due to the fact that the wounds are deep and the natural tendency of the deeper, divided structures is to separate, thereby interfering with skin healing and approximation. Proper application of adhesive plaster will often considerably lower the time necessary for healing.

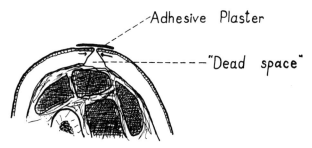

Figure 421

   The deeper wounds may have the following appearance on gross and cross section. (See Figs. 419, 420.)

   If a short strip of adhesive, such as the butterfly, is applied to this type of wound, then only the skin edges will be approximated, leaving considerable "dead space" below, in which blood, lymph, and serum may collect and thereby interfere with healing. (See Fig. 421.) However, if a longer piece of adhesive is applied, there is produced a greater tendency for the deeper structures to become approximated, thereby eliminating the "dead space" and favoring the healing process. (See Figs. 422, 423.) The direction of the lines of force illustrate how the deeper structures are forced together.

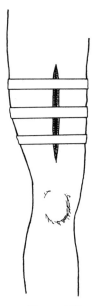

Figure 422

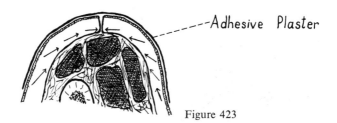

Figure 423

To aid further in forcing the deeper structures together, two tongue depressors may be rolled in several thicknesses of gauze and fixed to the skin, one on each side of the wound, by means of adhesive tape. These are referred to as *snubbers*. Thus, when the compressing strips of adhesive plaster are supplied, the tongue depressors tend to force the deeper structures together. (See Figs. 424, 425.)

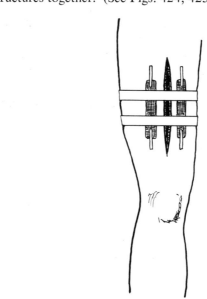

Figure 424

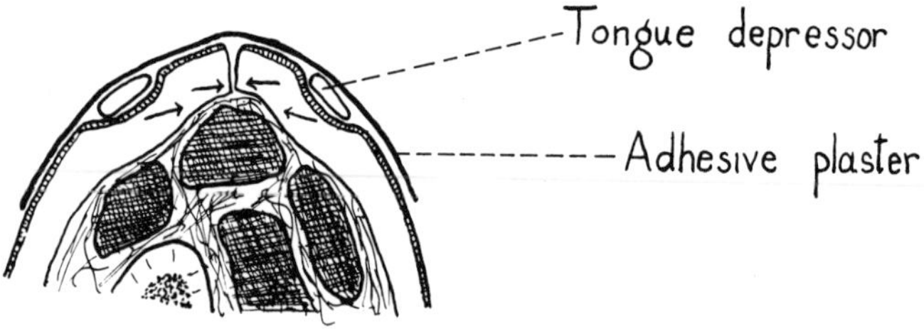

Figure 425

Adhesive Plaster Immobilization (*taping*)

Adhesive plaster, because of its firmness of application, is often used for immobilization and support of various parts of the body. Although it does not immobilize a part as well as does plaster of Paris, adhesive plaster does limit the motion of a part and support it, at the same time allowing a certain amount of function of the part. Thus, in strains and sprains, adhesive supports the part and limits its motion; however, it does allow a certain amount of activity. In some fractures, such as those of the ribs, adhesive plaster may be the only form of immobilization necessary. Where support is desired, and a still greater amount of activity is allowable, Elastoplast® or Peg® bandages may be used. These limit the motion of the parts, however, because of their elasticity, allow for a greater range of guarded motion.

Taping or *strapping* are the names often given to the procedure of immobilization with the aid of adhesive plaster. Numerous methods have been described for *taping* practically every part of the body; however, only the most commonly used procedures will be described here. A knowledge of these will make it possible for one to tape most any other part of the body.

These include: (a) Taping the ankle; (b) taping the knee; (c) taping the back, and (d) taping the chest.

It is highly recommended that particularly in taping, where the adhesive plaster is applied with considerable tension for a prolonged period, special attention be given to the preparation of the skin as described earlier in the chapter.

1. **Taping the Ankle:** The ankle is one of the most commonly traumatized joints, with injuries varying from slight *twists* to the more severe sprains. Adhesive plaster, properly applied, immobilizes the joint, supports it, and, at the same time, makes it possible for the patient to walk on the injured extremity.

Various methods have been described for taping the ankle; however, the Gibney strapping, in use for close to 50 years, has stood the test of time and use. Except for slight modifications of the original, the basic principles of most all of the methods are essentially the same. These comprise the application of alternating vertical and horizontal strips of adhesive plaster to the lower leg, foot, and ankle.

Directions

It is best to have the patient sitting on a table or edge of a high bed, with the injured foot hanging down. This makes it easier for the surgical dresser, and allows for more efficient application of the dressing. The foot is held in slight dorsiflexion by the patient. A long strip of gauze is so placed that the center passes around the toes of the foot, while the patient holds the two ends as he would a pair of reins. By this means he can hold the foot at any angle desired by the dresser. If the injury is over the lateral aspect of the ankle, the foot should be taped in slight eversion. If it is over the medial aspect, the foot should be taped in slight inversion. These positions allow for better healing of the injured parts. Strips of adhesive, 1 inch wide, are used throughout.

A. The first strip is vertical. Beginning on the dorsolateral aspect of the leg, at the junction of the middle and lower thirds, bring the adhesive down along the Achilles tendon, posterior to the lateral malleolus, around and under the heel, up along the foot posterior to the medial malleolus, again along the Achilles tendon, up to the level of the starting point. (See Fig. 426.)

B. The second strip is horizontal. Beginning at the outer border of the foot, near the fifth toe, carry the adhesive strip around

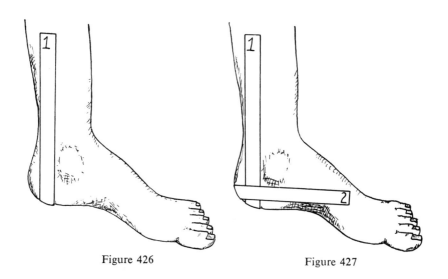

Figure 426   Figure 427

the lower part of the back of the heel, and end it on the medial aspect of the foot, over the first metatarsal bone. (See Fig. 427.)

C. The third strip is vertical, and is applied just anterior to the first strip, overlapping the latter by ½ inch. It follows a course similar to that of the first strip. (See Fig. 428.)

D. The fourth strip is horizontal, and is applied just superior to the second strip, overlapping the latter by ½ inch. (See Fig. 429.)

E. The fifth strip is vertical. (See Fig. 430.)

F. The sixth strip is horizontal. (See Fig. 431.)

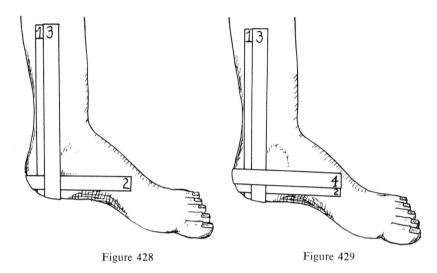

Figure 428   Figure 429

Approximately six vertical and six horizontal strips will adequately cover the ankle. Additional strips may be used, as indicated by the size of the part. (See Figs. 432, 433, 434.) The horizontally applied strips should not completely encircle the foot, since such application may constrict the circulation of the foot. The upper borders of the vertical strips may be fixed in place with a partially circular strip of adhesive one inch wide. (See Fig. 435.) A roller gauze bandage may be applied over the entire adhesive plaster dressing to fix the latter more firmly in place.

2. **Taping the Knee:** Adhesive plaster immobilization of the knee joint is utilized for a wide variety of purposes, including both traumatic and nontraumatic disease. Strains, sprains, and certain stages of arthritis are only a few of the many indications for strapping the knee. The adhesive strips must extend from below the tibial tubercle to well above the upper border of the patella, so that the entire overlying surface of the capsule of the joint and quadriceps bursa is covered.

Directions

Two-inch-wide strips of adhesive are used. These are applied in a basket weave fashion.

A. Begin strip No. 1 on the lateral aspect of the leg, about 3 inches below the level of the tibial tubercle, and carry it diagonally upward, across the tibial tubercle to the medial aspect of the leg. This first strip should encircle the leg for a distance of slightly more than half its diameter. (See Fig. 436.)

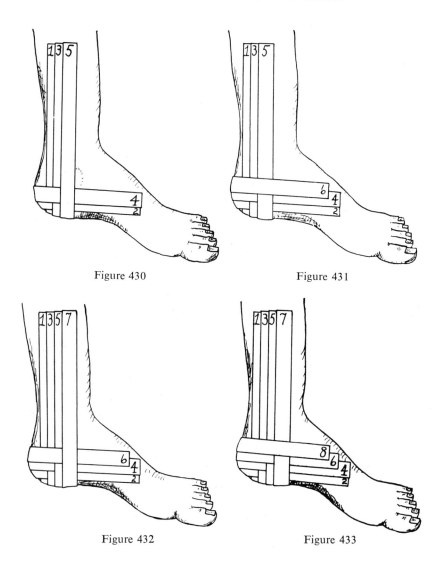

Figure 430

Figure 431

Figure 432

Figure 433

B. Apply strip No. 2 in a fashion similar to strip No. 1; however, begin on the medial aspect of the leg, carry it across the tibial tubercle and finish on the lateral aspect of the leg. Thus, strip No. 2 crosses strip No. 1, over the tibial tubercle. (See Fig. 437.)

C. Strip No. 3 is exactly similar to strip No. 1, except that it is applied slightly higher than No. 1, overlapping the latter for a distance of one inch. (See Fig. 438.)

D. Strip No. 4 is similar to strip No. 2, except that it overlaps the latter for a distance of one inch. (See Fig. 439.)

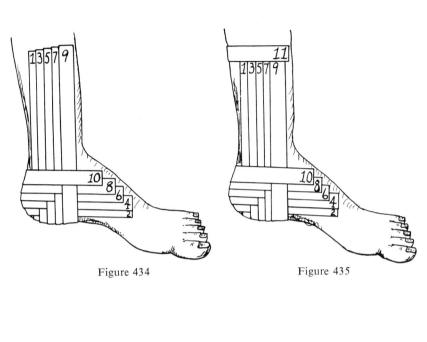

Figure 434   Figure 435

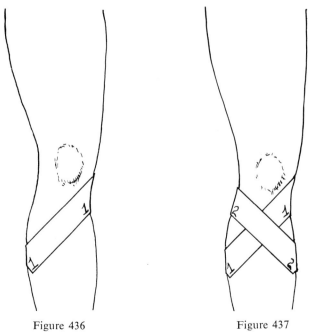

Figure 436   Figure 437

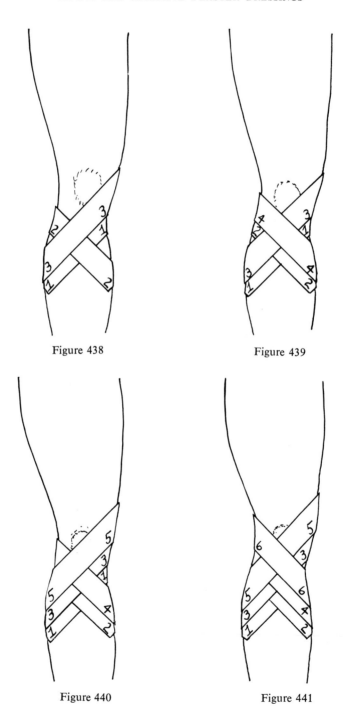

Figure 438

Figure 439

Figure 440

Figure 441

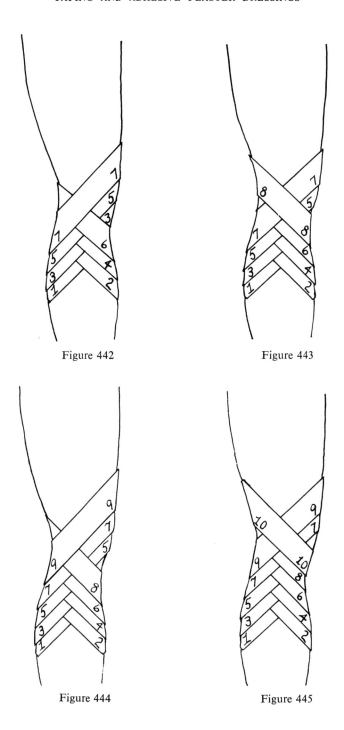

Figure 442

Figure 443

Figure 444

Figure 445

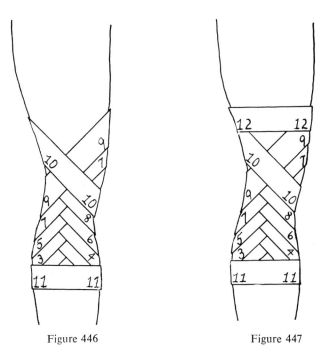

Figure 446   Figure 447

E. Strips Nos. 5, 6, 7, etc., are applied in a similar fashion, alternating first lateral to medial, and then medial to lateral, until the entire knee is covered. (See Figs. 440, 441, 442, 443, 444, 445.)

F. Finally, apply two transverse horizontal strips, one at the upper border, the other at the lower border of the diagonal strips. (See Figs. 446, 447.)

It must be remembered that none of the strips should completely encircle the limb, as this may interfere with the circulation. The entire dressing may then be covered with a roller gauze bandage, to hold it more firmly in place.

3. **Taping the Back:** A wide variety of strains and sprains involves the muscles, ligaments, and joints of the lumbar, sacral, and iliac regions. Many of these require adhesive plaster immobilization. Fractures of the transverse processes of the vertebrae are usually treated with adhesive plaster immobilization. Numerous methods have been devised for strapping the back. Basically, these are practically all the same.

Directions

Strips of adhesive, 3 or 4 inches wide and 18 to 20 inches long, are used.

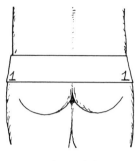
Figure 448

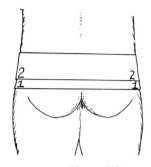
Figure 449

A. Apply one of the strips just above and anterior to the trochanter of the femur on one side, and draw it tightly across the lower back to a point above the opposite trochanter. (See Fig. 448.)

B. Apply a second strip, similar to the first, above and overlapping the latter by 2 inches. (See Fig. 449.)

C. Apply a third strip, above and overlapping the second strip by 2 inches. (See Fig. 450.)

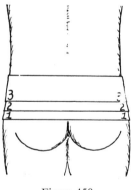
Figure 450

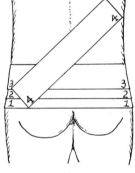
Figure 451

D. Apply a diagonal strip, which crosses upward from one side of the back to the other. This strip begins at the level of the first two horizontal strips. (See Fig. 451.)

E. Apply a similar diagonal strip, from the opposite side of the back. (See Fig. 452.)

F. Proceed upward on the back with alternating diagonal strips, until the lower back is well covered. (See Figs. 453, 454, 455, 456.)

G. Terminate the dressing with a transverse horizontal strip across the diagonal strips. (See Fig. 457.)

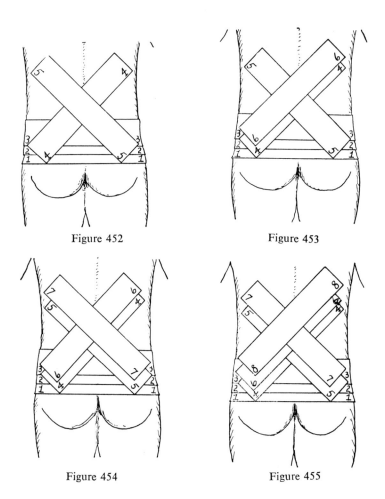

Figure 452

Figure 453

Figure 454

Figure 455

4. **Taping the Chest:** The chest is frequently immobilized for both traumatic and nontraumatic involvement. Noncomplicated fractures of the ribs are treated solely with adhesive plaster immobilization. For pleurisy and painful respiration, adhesive plaster immobilization is an excellent adjunct to other forms of therapy. The most common error in strapping the chest is the use of adhesive strips which are not sufficiently long.

Directions

Prepare several strips of adhesive plaster, three inches wide, and long enough to encircle about three-quarters of the circumference of the chest. Instruct the patient to raise the arm of the side to be immobilized,

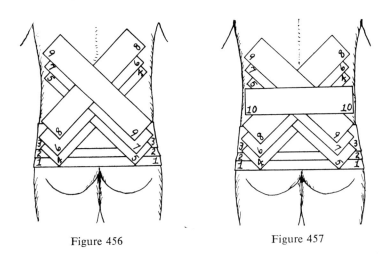

Figure 456 Figure 457

above his head. He is instructed to breathe deeply and, at the end of an
expiration, is told to hold his breath. At this point, the first strip of
adhesive plaster is applied. He is instructed to breathe several times and
then to hold his breath again at the end of an expiration. The second
strip is then applied. Subsequent strips are similarly applied.

Assume the right half of the chest is to be immobilized.

A. Beginning at the left border of the sternum, apply the first
strip of adhesive across the sternum, the front of the right chest,
around the right side and on to the back of the right chest, across
and beyond the midline of the back, well on to the left side of the
back for a distance of at least 4 or 5 inches. (See Figs. 458, 459.)

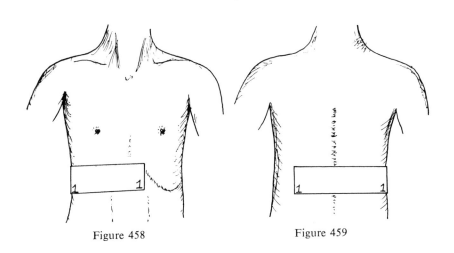

Figure 458 Figure 459

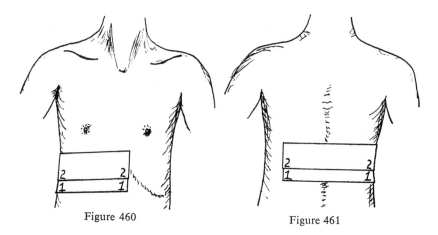

Figure 460   Figure 461

B. Apply the subsequent strips, from below upward, over the same course, each strip overlapping the preceding one for a distance of 1½ to 2 inches. (See Figs. 460, 461, 462, 463, 464, 465.)

Apply a gauze dressing over the nipple to protect it from the plaster. (See Fig. 462.)

Occasionally, to fix the adhesive plaster more firmly, a wide roller bandage, 6 inches wide, or a wide binder may be applied over the adhesive plaster.

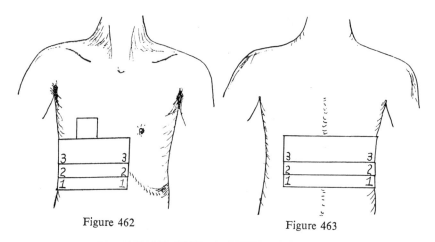

Figure 462   Figure 463

In strapping a chest for pleurisy, it is important to apply the first strip partly below the level of the costal margin. In this manner the ribs of the costal margin are well immobilized, this being the most effective means of preventing expansion of a side of the chest.

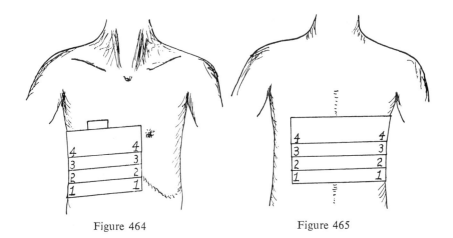

Figure 464   Figure 465

Skin Traction in the Treatment of Fractures: Traction upon the skin is one of the commonly employed forms of maintaining traction in the treatment of some fractures, as well as in a variety of muscle and joint disease conditions. Adhesive plaster is firmly applied to the skin, and then roller gauze or other bandages are applied around the adhesive to fix it more securely. It is important to prepare the skin adequately in such application, since traction exposes the skin to considerable trauma and strain. (See *Preparation of skin,* earlier in this chapter.) For traction, it is preferable to use the specially prepared adhesives. Made with moleskin or similar back cloth, these give firm support, are less likely to stretch, and, in addition, afford a rough surface upon which the gauze roller bandage will not slip. (See Fig. 466, *Spiral application of adhesive tape for traction.*)

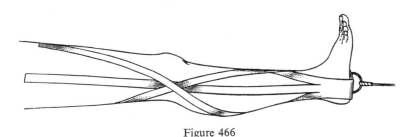

Figure 466

Adhesive Plaster in the Support of Bivalved Casts: After plaster-of-Paris casts are bivalved, adhesive plaster strips are employed to hold the plaster parts in place. (See Fig. 467.)

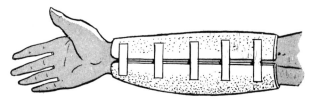

Figure 467

Adhesive Plaster in the Epithelialization of Wounds: In clean granulating wounds, particularly those following burns, in which the epithelium is gone, adhesive plaster may be used to encourage epithelialization. Narrow strips, one-half inch wide, are placed in bridgelike fashion across the wound. These should first be flamed prior to application. The epithelium tends to grow along the borders of the adhesive. (See Fig. 468.)

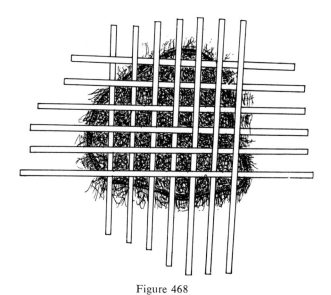

Figure 468

6. REMOVAL OF ADHESIVE PLASTER

Following the removal of adhesive plaster, two things are often noticed. In some areas, portions of the adhesive material come free from the back cloth and remain attached to the skin. This material may easily be removed from the skin by rubbing with a piece of gauze moistened with either benzene or ether. Following the use of benzene, the excess fluid should be removed with alcohol. In other areas, raw surfaces of the skin are present, the epidermis having become denuded. These areas are quite tender and a source of discomfort to the patient, and, in addition, may be a focus of secondary infection.

Careful observation has revealed that these raw surfaces are often the result of improper removal of the adhesive plaster. Over the extremities, where the skin is thick and firm, the common practice of removing strips of adhesive with a sudden jerk usually is unattended by any undesirable results. However, over the chest and abdomen, where the skin is more delicate, sudden jerking away of the adhesive tends to carry away some of the upper layers of the skin, leaving the denuded areas. It is recommended that over these more tender areas, the skin be carefully peeled away from the adhesive. Thus, the adhesive is held firmly in one hand, while the other hand gently pushes the skin away from the plaster.

To facilitate the removal of adhesive plaster, the entire back cloth may be moistened with ether or benzene.

In removing adhesive from wounds in which the plaster is used directly over the wound to approximate the skin surfaces, or used over gauze dressings, care must be taken not to pull the healing wound edges apart. Thus, the adhesive should be removed toward the wound, rather than away from it. The two ends should be freed first, and the portions over the wound last.

Following removal of adhesive plaster, the area should be gently dabbed with alcohol (70 per cent) on a sponge. If there is considerable raw surface, the application of alcohol may be too painful, and thus a one per cent solution of mercurochrome may be substituted. Talcum powder may then be applied to render a pleasant, cooling sensation. When adhesive plaster must be reapplied to an area from which it has just been removed, it is advisable to apply at least two to three coats of mercurochrome prior to application. Denuded areas should first be covered with small pieces of vaseline gauze and then dry gauze. The adhesive is then placed over these.

UNIT SIX ...

SPLINTS

On Splints

Ambrose Paré, one of the greatest surgeons in France in the 17th Century, when suffering from a fractured leg, instructed his friend, Richard Hubert, who attended him, as follows:

"You must fortify the sides of my limb with junks made of tents or little sticks, and lined with linen cloth."

CONTENTS OF UNIT SIX

Splints

Chapter 25
Basic Principles and Standard Splints

Chapter 26
Emergency Splinting of Fractures

25

Basic Principles and Standard Splints

---

1. Introduction—Definition and uses of splints.
2. Fractures.
3. Anatomicophysiological considerations.
4. Materials used for splints.
5. Qualities of a good splint.
6. Regional application of splints for fractures.

---

1. INTRODUCTION: DEFINITION AND USES OF SPLINTS

A splint may be defined as any piece of wood, metal, plastic, or other material for keeping the fragments of a fractured bone, or other movable part, in a state of rest. Exclusive of fractures, other indications for the use of splints include:

(a) Recently reduced dislocations in which the surrounding tissues have not had time to heal;

(b) infectious arthritis, in which movement of the joints may lead to considerable pain;

(c) operative cases in which the muscles, tendons, or skin have been repaired and in which movement, prior to adequate healing, may lead to disruption of the sites of repair;

(d) congenital abnormalities which may be improved by proper alignment and position of the parts; and

(e) temporary support of extremities in which there has been partial loss of function resulting from nutritional or metabolic disturbances.

It will not be the purpose of this chapter to dwell upon each of the above uses of splints; nor will an attempt be made to present the methods of diagnosis and treatment of all of the fractures in the body, with an expression of preference for any particular method. This is left to the more thorough and comprehensive texts devoted to this subject; however, an attempt will be made to present the anatomy of some of the more common fractures in the body, and the basic principles involved in the use of splints for emergency, and subsequent therapy in these as well as other fractures. A working knowledge of the application of splints for fractures would make it possible for one to utilize splints for most of the other uses already enumerated.

2. FRACTURES

A fracture may be defined as a break in the continuity of a bone, either partial or complete. The two main types of fractures are:

The *simple,* in which the fragments of bone have not broken through the skin; and

The *compound,* in which there is a communication between the fractured surfaces of bone and the surface of the body. It may be made by the sharp end of a fractured bone which penetrates the skin, or by a bullet which passes in from the outside, fracturing the bone.

The diagnosis of a compound fracture is relatively simple, particularly if the fragments of bone protrude through an opening in the skin. The simple fracture, however, is not always so readily diagnosed. The important signs and symptoms of fracture are:

Deformity of the part, due to displacement of the bone fragments and the soft tissues.

Abnormal mobility, due to the break in continuity of the bone and failure to function as a unit.

Crepitus, or grating sensation, which is produced by the rubbing upon each other of the rough ends of the fragments.

Loss of function, which may be due to pain, weakness, or actual loss of mechanical support.

Pain, which is elicited by direct pressure over the fracture site, or by attempt to move the part.

Swelling.

Bleb formation, resulting from extensive hemorrhage and ecchymosis.

3. ANATOMICO-PHYSIOLOGICAL CONSIDERATIONS

The care and treatment of fractures would be a relatively simple matter if one had to be concerned with only the fractured bones. Of probably greater significance in a fracture is the associated injury to the soft tissues, including the muscles, tendons, nerves, arteries, veins, and lymphatics. In a simple fracture in which a bone is merely cracked, with no displacement of the fragments, the soft tissue injury may be minimal, and this only as a result of local edema and hemorrhage; however, fractures in which the bony fragments are displaced from their normal alignment may lead to considerable injury to the surrounding soft tissues. The greater the degree of displacement, the sharper and more jagged the edges of the fractured bones, and the closer the bones are to vital structures, the greater would be the possibility for soft tissue damage. Following a fracture, the muscles of the part tend to contract and go into spasm. This leads to greater displacement and further wedging of the fractured fragments into the soft tissues with resultant increased damage. Careless movement of a fractured bone, without comprehensive knowledge of the basic anatomical and physiological structure, may equally lead to unnecessary soft tissue damage.

One of the basic principles in all surgical dressing and bandaging is *respect for living tissues,* with an attempt to avoid the superimposition of additional trauma to damage already done. At the time of occurrence of a fracture, a certain amount of soft tissue injury occurs. If it were possible to treat the fracture immediately at the site of injury, the soft tissue injury could be reduced to a minimum. Unfortunately, this is rarely possible, and thus the patient must be transported from the site of injury to either a hospital or physician's office. It is in this transportation that anatomico-physiological structure is of greatest importance. The injured part must be immobilized, that is, maintained at rest, in the most favorable position for the prevention of soft tissue injury. Splints are utilized for this immobilization, their function being twofold: (a) to prevent movement of the injured fragments of bone, and (b) to overcome and prevent further muscular spasm from forcing the fragments of bone into the neighboring soft tissues. It might be added that after reduction of a fracture, splints or other methods of immobilization are applied for the same purpose, namely: (a) to allow the bone to heal by keeping the injured fragments at rest and in proper apposition, and (b) to prevent muscle spasm from moving the fragments out of position.

The immobilization of the fragments of fractured bones and the control of muscle spasm are based on the principle of *fixed traction.* This may be defined as traction or force exerted on the end of a limb, pulling against, or away from a fixed point at the base of the limb where it joins the body. This fundamental method is frequently applied in the treatment of those fractures in which the fragments of bone, even after reduction, tend to become displaced as a result of muscle spasm. A more detailed discussion of the application of *fixed traction* will be presented in the next chapter, under *Emergency Splinting of Fractures.*

4. MATERIALS USED FOR SPLINTS

A wide variety of materials has been utilized for splints, the most commonly used ones being: (a) wood; (b) metal; (c) plaster of Paris; (d) plastics, and (e) cardboard.

Some of these materials, such as wood, metal, and plastics, are obtainable in ready-prepared form for immediate application; however, inability to obtain any of these specially prepared materials should not prevent one from adequately immobilizing a fractured bone. The number of other materials and objects capable of serving as splints is innumerable and here the ingenuity of the surgical dresser comes to the fore. Tennis racquets, baseball bats, canes, crutches, umbrellas, shovels, broomsticks, newspapers, pillows, and golf clubs are only a few of the objects which, properly applied, may adequately serve as splints. These objects are for the most part of temporary value in immobilization. For permanent therapeutic immobilization, there are two main methods:

The Application of Plaster-of-Paris Dressing

Following reduction of many fractures, plaster of Paris is applied and immobilization is thereby obtained. The main advantage of this method is that the plaster may be molded into any desired form or shape.

The Use of Various Types of Mechanical Apparatus and Metal Splints

A wide variety of well padded metal splints has been commercially prepared for practically every type of fracture in the body. These are light, durable, and so constructed as to treat the fractures on a sound anatomicophysiological basis. In the presentation of the various fractures, illustrations of these splints will serve to demonstrate the fundamental principles of therapy, as well as the correct anatomical position of the parts for proper alignment of the fractured parts.

5. QUALITIES OF A GOOD SPLINT

A good splint must have certain features to be of value. These are:

It must serve its purpose and function well; that is, it must be of adequate size, density, consistency, and strength to maintain a particular part at rest.

It must be capable of being applied and removed quickly, easily, and with a minimum of discomfort to the patient.

It must be light weight and comfortable for the patient.

It should not be excessive in cost.

It should be capable of maintaining the part in complete immobilization from the time of injury to the time when the patient may begin activity of the part.

It should be permeable to X-rays so that roentgenograms may be taken from time to time without necessitating the removal of the splint.

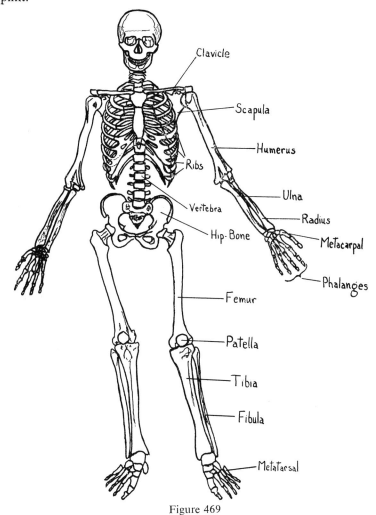

Figure 469

6. REGIONAL APPLICATION OF SPLINTS FOR FRACTURES

This section will be devoted to a presentation of some of the most commonly encountered fractures. Wherever possible, the anatomical changes resulting from fracture will be illustrated. It will then become evident why muscle spasm is of such significance in the displacement of fragments. The various splints for each of these fractures will be illustrated as well. It is hoped that from the illustrations of the deformity and displacement following fracture and the corrected position as shown in the splint, one will see the rationale of the methods of therapy in the various fractures. In addition, one should appreciate along which lines emergency treatment should be directed, so as to produce minimal displacements of fragments and minimal soft tissue damage.

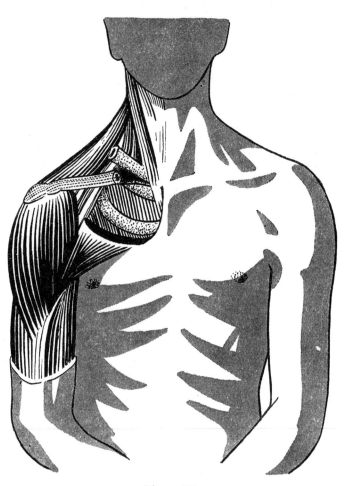

Figure 470

Fracture of the Clavicle

The clavicle, or collarbone, forms the anterior portion of the shoulder girdle. It is attached to the sternum medially, and is the only bony connection between the upper extremity and the trunk. It serves to hold the shoulder upward, outward, and backward. Beneath the clavicle, the various arteries, veins, and nerves pass from the neck into the axilla and arm. In fracture of the clavicle, the entire shoulder girdle, that is, the scapula and the upper extremity, drop downward, forward, and inward. The lateral fragment of bone may compress the brachial plexus and axillary vessels, although severe injury to these soft structures is rare. (See Fig. 470.) The treatment must, therefore, consist of correcting the position by lifting and pulling the arm and shoulder upward, outward, and backward. It is best to get both shoulders into the corrected position. This prevents undue stress on the injured side. This may be accomplished by various means, which include:

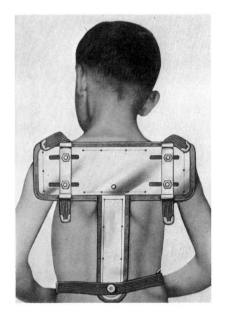

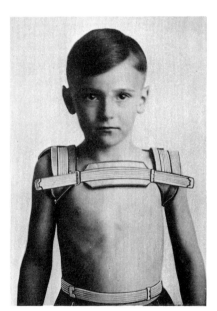

Figure 471   Figure 472

The clavicular cross (See Figs. 471, 472), the strap splint (See Figs. 473, 474), and the figure-of-eight bandage of both shoulders.

The last is made with gauze, muslin, or plaster of Paris, the dressing simulating the strap splint in structure. (See Figs. 473, 474.)

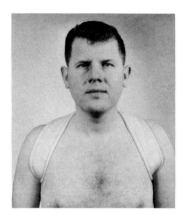

Figure 473

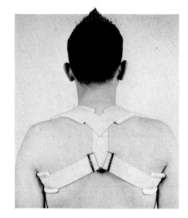

Figure 474

Fracture of the Humerus

The humerus, or arm bone, is subject to a wide variety of fractures, classified on the basis of site of fracture. The degrees of displacement and deformity are directly related to the relationship between fracture site and location of muscle insertion. Thus, in a fracture through the surgical neck of the humerus, the upper fragment is abducted and externally rotated by those muscles attached to it. These include the supraspinatus, the infraspinatus, and the teres minor muscles. The lower fragment is adducted by the pectoralis major and the teres major muscles. These opposing forces tend to cause considerable displacement of the fragments. (See Fig. 475.)

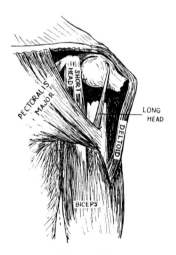

Figure 475

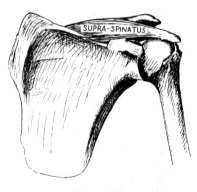

Figure 476

In fractures through the greater tuberosity of the humerus, the supra-spinatus tends to displace the tuberosity upward. (See Fig. 476.)

The ideal positions for alignment of the fragments in each of these fractures is abduction. The effect of such abduction is presented in the following illustrations (See Figs. 477, 478.) The so-called *airplane splint* is used for these types of fracture since it efficiently maintains the arm in abduction. This splint transmits the weight of the abducted arm to the trunk and the pelvis. (See Figs. 479, 480.)

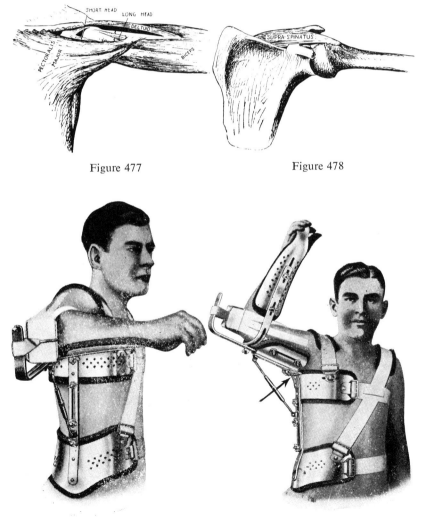

Figure 477   Figure 478

Figure 479   Figure 480

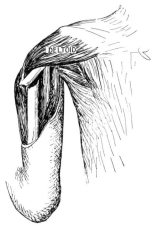 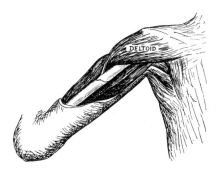

Figure 481   Figure 482

Splints of this shape may be made of a right triangle arrangement of several strips of wood, or heavy cardboard, or even plaster of Paris; however, the metal splint is so constructed as to allow for a greater degree of adjustment and regulation.

Fractures through the shaft of the humerus tend to result in abduction of the upper fragment due to the action of the deltoid muscle. (See Fig. 481.) This can be corrected by producing abduction of the entire arm, with the application of traction. (See Fig. 482.) The ideal splint for treatment of fracture of the shaft of the humerus is the Robert Jones splint. (See Figs. 483, 484.) This splint is useful for traction and countertraction (fixed traction) on the humerus, and also for support of the forearm.

Fracture of the shaft of the humerus is one of the most important fractures from the viewpoint of soft tissue damage. The radial nerve, which supplies the extensor muscles of the forearm and hand, winds around and is in close approximation to the shaft of the humerus. It can readily be injured either in the process of fracture, or in the careless manipulation of the fragments. The proximity of the nerve to the bony fragments is illustrated. (See Fig. 485.)

Fracture of the Elbow

Fracture of the elbow often refers to the olecranon process of the ulna. The triceps muscle tends to pull the upper fragment upward. (See Fig. 486.) Approximation of the fragments may be produced by the position of extension. (See Fig. 487.)

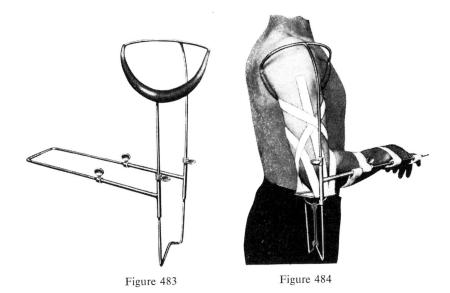

Figure 483   Figure 484

Fracture of Radius: Colles' Fracture

This fracture involves the lower 4 cm. of the radius, and produces what is often referred to as the "silver fork deformity," the lower forearm and wrist assuming the shape of a fork. (See Figs. 488, 489.)

The most significant feature in this type of fracture is the possible injury to the flexor tendons of the forearm and hand, which in this fracture are both stretched and in close approximation to the fractured ends of bone. (See Fig. 489.) It is obvious here why one cannot overemphasize the importance of careful manipulation of a fracture. Following reduction of this fracture, the hand and forearm may be immobilized in a Colles splint. (See Fig. 490.)

Fractures of Metacarpal Bones

The metacarpals comprise the bony framework of the palm and dorsum of the hand. Simple fractures of these bones with little or no displacement are easily treated by simple immobilization. Variations in types of fractures may produce varying degrees of deformity. In these, methods of reduction and immobilization will depend on the degrees of deformity produced by the angle of fracture and muscular contractions and spasm. Following reduction of some of these fractures, a metacarpal splint may be used. (See Fig. 491.)

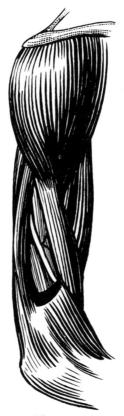

Figure 485

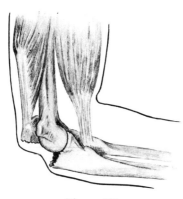

Figure 486

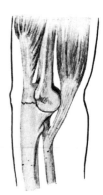

Figure 487

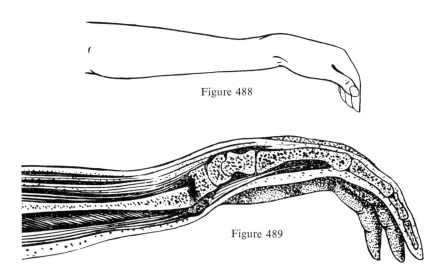

Figure 488

Figure 489

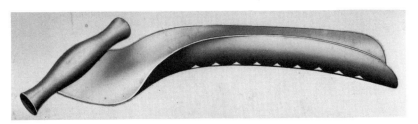

Figure 490

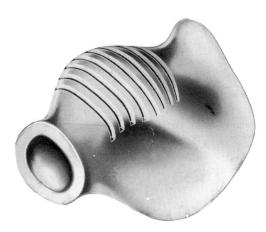

Figure 491

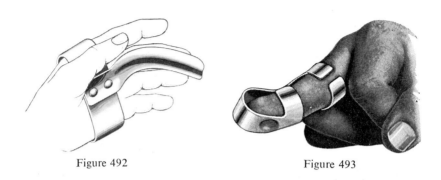

Figure 492   Figure 493

Fractures of the Phalanges

Fractures of the phalanges may be of various types. In simple fractures which require immobilization in the normal or neutral position of the fingers, metallic or tongue depressor splints may be used. (See Fig. 492.)

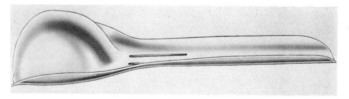

Figure 494

A common injury is the *baseball finger,* in which there is a fracture of the distal phalanx, with inability to extend the terminal phalanx. A special splint immobilizes the finger in hyperextension. (See Fig. 493.) This same deformity may result from a laceration of the extensor tendon of the finger at the level of the distal interphalangeal joint. In such cases, the same method of immobilization may be used as for the fracture.

One of the most commonly used splints for a wide variety of hand wounds, infections, and injuries, is the Mason-Allen Universal hand splint. (See Fig. 494.) This allows the hand to rest in the *position of function.* In this position the wrist is maintained in slight dorsiflexion. The finger joints are all in slight flexion. The thumb is in abduction, midway between pronation and supination.

Fractures of the Femur

The femur, the largest bone in the body, has acting upon it some of the most powerful muscles in the body. Thus, in fractures involving this long bone, there is a tendency for muscular spasm to cause a considerable displacement and overriding of the fragments. The iliopsoas, attached to the lesser trochanter, tends to cause flexion and external rotation of the upper fragment in fractures through the upper part of the shaft of the femur. (See Fig. 495.)

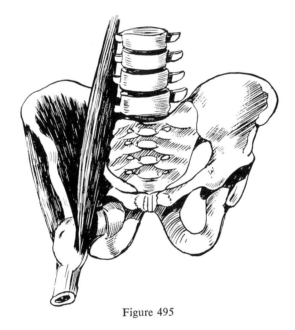

Figure 495

In fractures through the lower third of the bone, the powerful calf muscles tend to cause posterior displacement of the lower fragment. (See Fig. 496.) It is important to note that in the latter fracture the popliteal vessels and nerves are specially prone to injury.

The great majority of fractures of the neck and shaft of the femur are treated by internal fixation by a wide variety of metallic appliances. Where this is not possible, or not indicated, reduction and immobilization are achieved by utilization of traction procedures.

Fractures of the femoral shaft are most commonly treated by flexing at the hip joint, so as to relax the spastic muscles. At the same time traction is applied to maintain the fragments in place and to overcome whatever muscle spasm still persists.

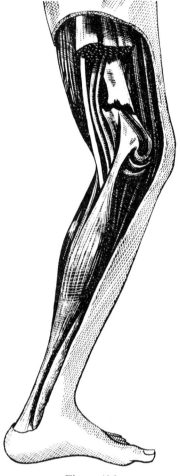

Figure 496

The most commonly used method of maintaining immobilization for these fractures is the *Russell traction* method, which combines suspension of the extremity and traction. (See Fig. 497.)

Fractures of the Leg and Ankle

A wide variety of fractures may involve the tibia, fibula, and ankle joint. Many of these require operative manipulation and immobilization with plaster of Paris. Others require open reduction and mechanical union of the fragments. Often following reduction, the leg is immobilized in leg splints, which are adaptable to any degree of flexion or extension. (See Fig. 498.)

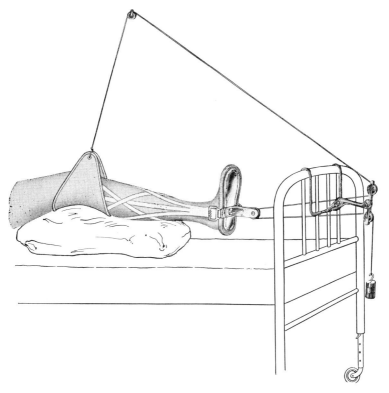

Figure 497

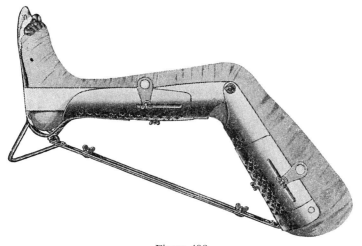

Figure 498

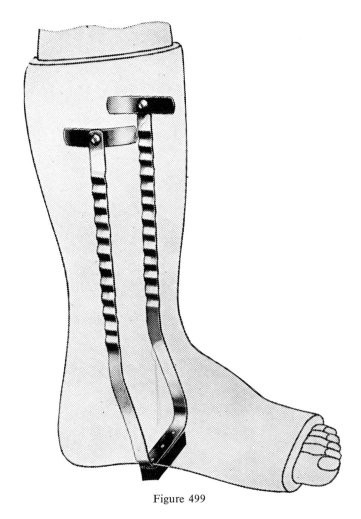

Figure 499

In various fractures of the ankle, it is possible to allow a patient to walk fairly easily and early, with the use of the so-called *walking splints*. These are incorporated into plaster-of-Paris casts and convey the weights of the body to the upper part of the leg, away from the foot. (See Fig. 499.)

Fractures of the Vertebral Column or Spine

Fractures of the spine are significant from two main viewpoints, namely: (a) Possible injury to the spinal cord, and (b) interference with or alteration of the normal posture of the individual.

Fractures involving the spinous processes or transverse processes of the vertebrae do not result in much soft tissue damage, and may be immobilized by simple adhesive plaster strapping; however, injuries to the vertebral bodies may very readily lead to flexion of the spine at the site of fracture with resultant spinal cord damage. (See Fig. 500.) Obviously, it is the acute flexion of the spine which produces the damage and thus the basic principle in treating vertebral column fractures is to maintain the body in a position of hyperextension. For cervical spine injuries, the neck may be prevented from flexing by means of the *cervical brace*. (See Fig. 501.) For maintaining hyperextension of the dorsal and lumbar spines, the *Taylor brace* is employed. (See Fig. 502.)

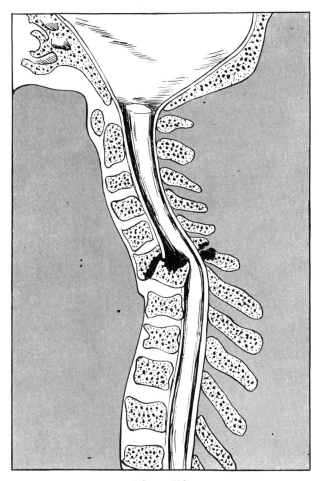

Figure 500

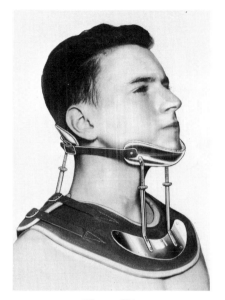

Figure 501

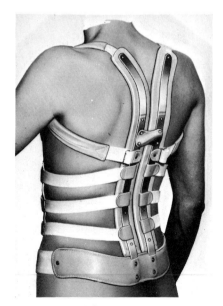

Figure 502

26

Emergency Splinting of Fractures

1. Introduction.
2. "Splint 'em where they lie."
3. Regional emergency application of splints.

1. INTRODUCTION

As was stressed in the previous chapter, fractures unfortunately cannot be adequately treated at the site of injury. The patient must be transported to either a hospital or a physician's office. It is this early transportation of the patient which plays a most important role in determining the degree of soft tissue damage, the length of the period of healing, and hospitalization, and, in the final analysis, the success or failure of subsequent therapy.

2. "SPLINT 'EM WHERE THEY LIE"

Simple as it sounds, this basic maxim expresses the keynote of successful transportation of fractures. One may cite the hypothetical case of a person who, while crossing the street, is struck by an automobile and sustains a simple fracture of the tibia and fibula.

The patient cannot walk and so the first instinct of bystanders is to carry him from the street onto the sidewalk, or to the nearest drug store. With one supporting his head and shoulders, and the other holding his ankles, he is carried onto the sidewalk. In lifting the injured leg by the ankle, the carrier displaces the fragments of bone. With each step, the jagged edges of bone are moved, thereby producing increased soft tissue damage. The muscles are torn, blood vessels and nerves are injured, and marked hemorrhage and edema are produced.

In stepping onto the curb, the carrier gives the injured leg a sudden jolt and one of the sharp ends of the bone breaks through the skin. The patient now has a compound fracture which is subject to infection and a prolonged period of healing. With each step that the patient is carried beyond this point, the dirt or grease on his clothing is carried further into the wound. In some cases, the patient is then hurriedly placed into an automobile and rushed to a nearby hospital. More injury is produced in the attempt to place him into a comfortable position in the automobile. By the time he reaches the hospital, the patient is in a much worse condition than he was immediately following his injury. In fact, more damage has probably been done in transporting him than was done by the initial injury.

Ideally, such a case would be treated somewhat differently. The patient would be allowed to remain at rest wherever the accident occurred. He would be covered with blankets or coats until the ambulance, or whatever first aid conveyance is available, had arrived. A splint would be applied in such fashion as to immobilize the fragments of bone and prevent muscle spasm. With the splint applied, the patient would be transported. With such procedure, soft tissue trauma is minimized and the conversion of a simple fracture into a compound fracture would be most unlikely.

Three other principles of importance must be considered in the proper emergency management of fractures. These are:

Treatment of Shock

For the layman, this is limited to keeping the patient comfortable, at rest, and warm, by means of blankets and coats. The ambulance surgeon, or other qualified person, will usually administer a hypodermic of one of the opiates to combat shock further.

Care of Compound Fractures

Proper care of such wounds cannot be adequately performed at the site of injury. It is best to pour some antiseptic, such as aqueous iodine, Betadine®, Zephiran®, or Mercurochrome®, over the wound and then apply a sterile dressing.

Control of Bleeding

Bleeding is best controlled by the application of a simple compression bandage directly over the site of bleeding.

If any doubt exists as to whether there is a fracture, it is best to treat the patient as though a fracture is present.

3. REGIONAL EMERGENCY APPLICATION OF SPLINTS

It must be remembered that although the types of splints herein described and presented are standard apparatus, there is a wide variety of moderately rigid substances, any one of which may be used as a splint. The variety of available materials is limited only by the ingenuity of the bandager.

The Extremities

The application of some form of fixed traction is the only effective means of transporting a patient with a fracture of one of the long bones of either the upper or lower extremity. As already described, fixed traction implies the application of a force at the end of an extremity, pulling against or away from a fixed point at the base of the limb where it joins the body. A typical device for maintaining fixed traction is the Thomas splint. This consists of a steel rod, bent in such a fashion as to accommodate an extremity. The upper ends of the bent rod are attached to a leather-padded ring. (See Fig. 503.) Instead of a full

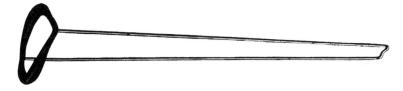

Figure 503

ring, there may be a half ring, the defect being replaced by a canvas strap, as in the Keller-Blake splint. (See Fig. 504.)

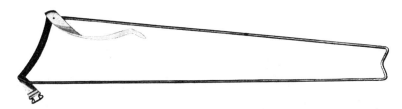

Figure 504

The Thomas splint obtains traction as follows: the ring is passed over the foot, knee, and thigh until it comes into contact with the ischial tuberosity. This represents the *fixed point* where the lower extremity meets the body. The two iron sides of the splint are now on each side of the extremity, with the end of the splint extending for a distance beyond the foot. The foot is then pulled down toward the end of the splint and firmly fixed with some form of hitch or buckle. In this manner, traction is exerted upon the entire lower extremity. (See Fig. 505.) This is the en-

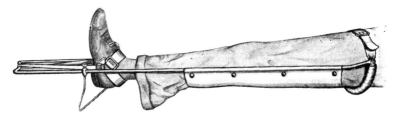

Figure 505

tire working principle of *fixed traction,* which is applicable to fractures of both lower and upper extremities. In the case of the latter, the axilla and shoulder are the fixed points for the application of the ring. The extremity should be suspended and supported by means of muslin, or special slings, between the two sides of the splint. (See Fig. 506.) It may be further immobilized by bandages which pass around both the extremity

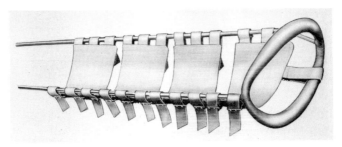

Figure 506

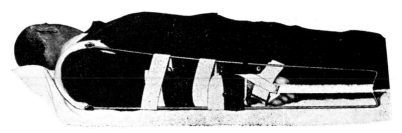

Figure 507

and the splint. A modification of the Thomas splint, with hinges at the junction of the ring and the rods, is applicable for maintaining fixed traction of the upper extremity. (See Fig. 507.)

The Steps in the Application of the Thomas Splint

Assuming a patient has a simple fracture of the femur, the following would be the steps in the application of a Thomas splint:

The patient is first treated for shock with blankets and morphine.

The Thomas splint is prepared by applying cotton wadding or other available material to the leather ring. This lessens the pressure on the ischial tuberosity.

Several slings are applied across the two rods, for support of the extremity. A towel may be suspended across the two rods and pinned in place. (See Fig. 506.) The splint is now ready for application.

The shoe of the injured extremity may be removed, or it may be allowed to remain in place. In fact, the latter is preferable since it protects the foot in the application of traction. An assistant grasps the foot with both hands and exerts a steady pull in the axis of the extremity. Once begun, this traction must be maintained until the splint traction is established.

While traction is being maintained, the entire extremity is lifted sufficiently off the ground to allow the ring to be passed over the foot, knee, and thigh to its resting point against the ischial tuberosity.

The ankle and foot are protected with cotton wadding and a traction hitch is applied to the ankle. This may be the ready prepared ankle hitch (See Fig. 505.) or a muslin bandage, applied in the form of a *Collins hitch.* (See Figs. 508, 509, 510, 511, 512, 513, 514.) This hitch is then attached to the end of the splint and tied firmly. A Spanish windlass made with a tongue depressor is then applied to the muslin bandage and the traction is increased by turning the tongue depressor. (See Figs. 514, 515.) When traction is adequate, the manual traction is released.

Several circular turns with a roller bandage are applied both above and below the knee, thus preventing anterior or lateral movement of the limb. The patient may now be moved, provided someone supports the splint.

The end of the splint is suspended by a rope from the roof of the ambulance or car and the patient transported thusly.

The Thomas splint is kept in position until some other form of traction or immobilization is ready to be applied.

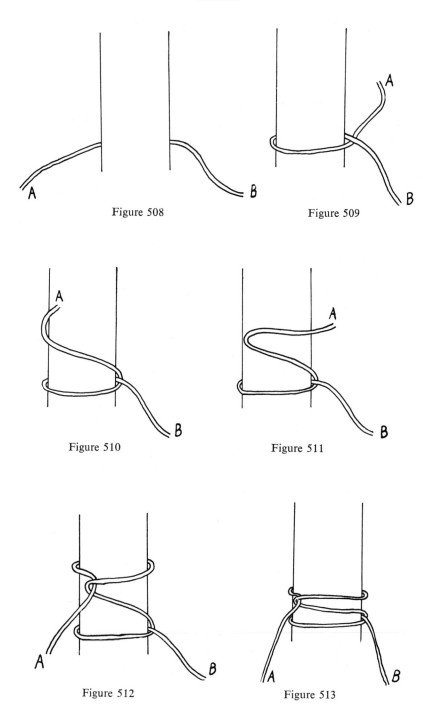

Figure 508

Figure 509

Figure 510

Figure 511

Figure 512

Figure 513

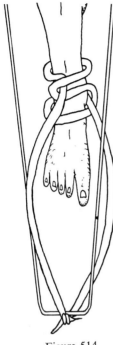
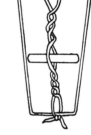

Figure 514   Figure 515

If splints of the Thomas type are not available, other methods for protecting the extremities may be utilized. The injured leg may be firmly bound to the uninjured leg, the latter acting as a splint. The entire extremity may be firmly fixed to a laterally placed board of wood or other rigid object.

In fractures of the humerus, where no splint is available, the arm may be firmly bound to the side of the chest, the forearm being supported in a sling which passes around the neck.

For splinting the tibia and fibula, basswood splints may be used. These consist of wide strips of a thin wood which are padded with cotton wadding and then applied to an extremity, one on the posterior, one on the medial, and one on the lateral aspect of the leg. A circular bandage holds these in place. A more effective modification of the basswood splint is the "coaptation splint," prepared from basswood splints and adhesive plaster. Several strips of basswood are applied side by side onto a wide strip of adhesive plaster. (See Fig. 516.) Longitudinal cuts are made in the basswood with a sharp knife. This makes for a splint which is flexible and can be molded quite easily to an extremity. (See Fig. 517.) A small splint of this type may be made with tongue depressors and adhesive plaster.

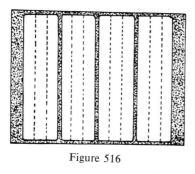

Figure 516

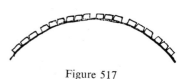

Figure 517

For fractures around the ankle, a pillow drawn tightly around the part serves as an excellent form of immobilization.

For fractures of the elbow, forearm, wrist, or hand, padded basswood splints or coaptation splints may be used. The forearm may be supported and splinted by flexing the elbow and pinning the sleeve of the injured forearm to the coat. Other splints may be prepared from folded newspapers, magazines, or any other rigid substances.

The Spine

As demonstrated in the previous chapter, the main danger in fractures of the spine is the possible injury to the spinal cord resulting from flexion of the vertebral column; thus, emergency splinting of the spine must be directed toward preventing flexion, and, if possible, obtaining hyperextension of the spine. The patient may be transported either on his back or in the prone position with his face down, depending upon the particular position in which he is found. Most important of all is the prevention of flexion. The ordinary stretcher constructed of a canvas suspended between two poles is not advisable for such injuries since it allows sagging of the back. A long, wide wooden board is an ideal stretcher for a patient with a spine injury. In lifting such a patient, at least three persons should be present, one to support his head and shoulders, one to support his lower extremities, and one to support the middle of his back. The patient must be moved as a unit, with absolutely no flexion of the spine. A good method of transporting such a patient is in the face-down position, on a long board, with a pillow under the face and one under the knees and thighs. In this manner, the spine is placed into a position of hyperextension. If transported on his back, the patient should have one or two pillows placed under the center of his back, allowing the head and buttocks to hang downward, thereby producing a moderate degree of hyperextension. In either method of transport, the patient should be firmly bound to the stretcher with roller bandages, or with triangles folded to cravats.

UNIT SEVEN ...

PLASTER-OF-PARIS DRESSINGS

27

Plaster-of-Paris Dressings

1. Introduction and purpose of immobilization.
2. Materials used:
   A. Essential characteristics.
   B. Types of materials.
   C. Plaster of Paris:
      (1) Chemistry.
      (2) Plaster-of-Paris bandages.
      (3) Care of plaster of Paris.
3. Preparation of the room and bed.
4. Preparation of the part to be immobilized:
   A. Cleansing.
   B. Padding.
5. Preparation and manipulation of the plaster-of-Paris bandage:
   A. Care of the hands.
   B. Dipping of the plaster bandages.
   C. Removal and compression of the bandage.
6. General rules and methods for application of plaster:
   A. Basic principles.
   B. Methods of application:
      (1) The circular cast:
         (a) *Smooth casts.*
         (b) *Window* in casts.
      (2) The molded splint:
         (a) Reinforcement of casts.
         (b) Maintenance of position of bone fragments.
7. Drying of plaster-of-Paris dressings.
8. Removal of plaster-of-Paris dressings.
9. The "soft" cast.

1. INTRODUCTION AND PURPOSE OF IMMOBILIZATION

Muslin bandages and adhesive plaster strappings are often utilized for the immobilization of various parts; however, there often arises the necessity for a greater degree of immobilization and support than is possible with either of these; thus, in the treatment of fractured bones and certain disease conditions of bones and joints, absolute immobilization and support are necessary for: (a) adequate healing of the bony parts; (b) prevention of injury to the tissues surrounding the injured or diseased bone; and (c) comfort of the patient.

Although the specific therapy for each type of fracture or disease condition of bone or joint is more adequately and thoroughly presented in books on surgery and orthopedics devoted to this purpose, it is well that the surgical dresser be thoroughly familiar with the basic materials and principles involved in the preparation of plaster-of-Paris dressings for immobilization.

2. MATERIALS USED

Essential Characteristics

A material must be used which, when applied, is soft, pliable, and can be easily adapted and molded to any part of the body. The material must have the power to harden to a firm, strong dressing, capable of holding a part immobilized in spite of any attempt to move it. It must dry quickly, else the bony parts may move out of the desired position before the dressing is firm and secure. The completed dressing should not be too heavy; otherwise, it may add to the discomfort of the patient.

Types of Materials

A survey of surgical literature reveals that a wide variety of substances has been used for immobilizing dressings. Hippocrates described a method of rubbing a softened wax into each turn of the bandage applied to a fractured extremity. When completed, the wax solidified and there was produced a firm dressing capable of immobilizing the part. This ancient method has been superseded by many more efficient and practical methods.

During the past few centuries, the following have been used: (a) Mixtures of wheat flour and whites of eggs; (b) mixtures of whites of eggs with powdered chalk; (c) mixtures of camphorated spirits, lead acetate, and egg whites; (d) dextrine, camphorated spirits, and water; and (e) plaster of Paris. At present, the most widely used substance is plaster of Paris. A plaster-of-Paris cast, or splint, properly applied, fits the part more accurately and is more comfortable than any other type of material or apparatus. Properly applied, a plaster dressing requires very little attention on the part of the surgeon until the time comes for its removal.

Plaster of Paris
Chemistry
Plaster of Paris, chemically, is gypsum or calcium sulfate which is crushed to a powder, and then deprived of 93 per cent of its water of crystallization by heating. The re-addition of water to the plaster of Paris results in a chemical union called *recrystallization* or *setting*. It is in this latter process that the plaster becomes hard. In addition, there is slight expansion of the plaster and the liberation of a moderate amount of heat. Once set, the plaster retains its shape indefinitely. It is possible, by varying the composition of the plaster, to alter the setting time of the plaster. The average setting time is seven minutes; however, there is fast setting plaster, which sets in three to six minutes, and slow setting plaster, which sets in 10 to 18 minutes. The addition of a small quantity of ordinary table salt to the water in which the plaster is immersed will shorten the time required for setting, but this is generally unnecessary.

Plaster-of-Paris Bandages
These are prepared by filling the meshes of a loosely woven material with the plaster and then rolling the material into the form of a roller bandage. The material used is crinoline, a loosely woven gauze, stiffened by starching. A piece of corrugated paper is often included in the middle of the roller bandage. This allows for more thorough penetration of the center of the roller when it is immersed in the water. The preparation of these bandages may be performed by hand or machine. The grades of plaster, the construction and degree of starching of the crinoline, and the distribution of the plaster in the handmade bandages may vary considerably. The hand preparation method is a slow process and these bandages have been replaced almost universally by the commercially prepared products. (See Fig. 518.)

Care of Plaster of Paris
It must be remembered that plaster of Paris, if exposed to the moisture in the air for any length of time, will readily take up some of this water of crystallization, set, and become lumpy. In this condition it is no longer of any value. For this reason the bandages are wrapped in a special moisture-proof paper and then kept in a closed box until ready for use. When not in use, the bandages should be kept well protected from the air in a cool, dry place.

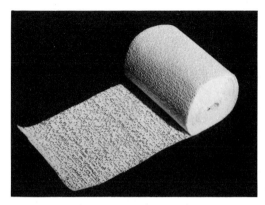

Figure 518

3. PREPARATION OF THE ROOM AND BED

In the operating room in which plaster is to be used, the floor should be covered with a sheet or cloth or newspaper. This prevents particles of plaster from adhering to the tile floors of the operating room.

When plaster is to be applied with the patient in bed, a sheet should be placed under the patient, if possible, thereby protecting the bed sheets, pillows, and blankets from the excess particles of plaster which fall in the process of application of the plaster. In the operating room as well, a sheet should be used to cover all blankets and sheets on the operating table, so that only the part to be dressed is exposed.

For the application of plaster, certain materials should always be available. These include a pail of water for dipping the plaster, a wooden board for unrolling the plaster, stockinet, cotton wadding, felt, plaster scissors, and a scalpel or other sharp knife.

4. PREPARATION OF THE PART TO BE IMMOBILIZED

Prior to the application of a plaster-of-Paris dressing, there must be proper and adequate preparation of the part with respect to (a) cleansing, and (b) padding.

Cleansing

The part is thoroughly cleansed with soap and water and then dried. It is then washed with either alcohol or ether, and dried again. Talcum powder is then applied. If considerable hair is present, the part should be shaved.

Padding

Although there are some surgeons who advocate and prefer skin-tight application of plaster with no padding, the majority of plaster dressings is applied over some underlying padding which is first applied to the skin. Tubular stockinet is first applied to the part. (See Fig. 21.) This is then covered with a layer of sheet cotton or cotton wadding, smoothly applied with spiral turns. Bony prominences, such as the elbow and the superior iliac spines, as well as nerves in close proximity to the skin, such as the ulnar and the peroneal, may all be further protected by the application of pieces of felt over the stockinet. In applying felt, it is important to bevel off the borders of the felt, otherwise these will cut into the skin and produce pressure sores. The importance of proper padding is appreciated when one realizes that inadequate padding may result in pressure necrosis of the skin as well as peripheral nerve involvement. Excessive padding leads to a loose-fitting cast, which does not immobilize the parts, is uncomfortable, and may also lead to pressure sores by excessive movement and irritation of the part.

5. PREPARATION AND MANIPULATION OF THE PLASTER-OF-PARIS BANDAGE

Care of the Hands

The bandager should wear rubber gloves or smear the hands with vaseline to prevent the plaster from adhering to the skin. If neither of these is used, the unpleasant harshness of the skin which the plaster causes is best remedied by rubbing the hands with a small amount of granulated sugar and then dissolving it upon the fingers with plain water. Vinegar may also be used to remove the adherent particles of plaster.

Dipping of the Plaster Bandages

The plaster bandage is immersed in a pail or basin of cold water until it ceases to yield bubbles of air which may be seen rising from the roller to the surface of the water. There is some controversy as to whether the bandage should be placed into the water on end, in a vertical position, or on its side, in a horizontal position. The objection to the vertical position is that more of the plaster may drop from the meshes of the material in this position. In favor of the vertical position is the belief that it allows for easier liberation of the air. Careful comparison and observation have revealed that two bandages, one in the vertical and the other in the horizontal position, immersed in water for the same length of time, have approximately the same degree of penetration of water, and the same degree of loss of plaster. Thus, bandages may be inserted into the water in either the vertical or horizontal position.

More important than the position, however, is the care with which the bandage is placed into the water, for carelessness in this phase of the procedure may result in considerable loss of plaster. It must be gently placed at the bottom of the pail or basin and not dropped into same. The bandage should not be disturbed while it is soaking in the water.

Removal and Compression of the Bandage

When the bandage is thoroughly saturated as indicated by the cessation of the bubbling, it should be removed from the water. This is done by inserting both hands into the water, grasping both ends of the roller, and removing it in this position. (See Fig. 519.) The surplus water is

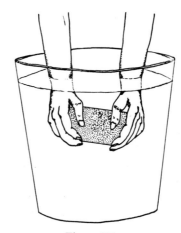

Figure 519

then removed by compressing the cylinder from end to end, toward the middle. Less plaster will be displaced by this method than by compressing the roller in the middle and forcing the water out of the ends. The degree to which the bandage is squeezed may vary with different surgeons, since some prefer to work with bandages which are quite wet, while others prefer them fairly dry.

It must be remembered that recrystallization of the plaster and hardening, or setting, takes place in the water as well as it does in the air, and thus a bandage allowed to remain in the water too long will *set* in fine particles like sand, rendering the bandage useless. If one person is applying the plaster, only one roller of bandage should be placed into the water at a time. When it is removed, another is inserted.

The person assisting the surgeon should unroll the bandage slightly in order to facilitate the task of the bandager, thereby saving time and effort.

6. GENERAL RULES AND METHODS FOR APPLICATION OF PLASTER

Basic Principles

Plaster-of-Paris bandages are applied with the same basic turns as are employed in the application of the ordinary gauze bandages, namely: (a) circular turns; (b) ascending and descending spiral turns; (c) recurrent turns; (d) figure-of-eight turns; and (e) spiral reverse turns.

The spiral reverse turns are not generally used, except where it is desired to alter, or reverse, the direction of a roller.

Following are several general rules which are of basic importance in the application of plaster dressings. Undoubtedly, numerous other suggestions will arise in the mind of the bandager as the scope of experience increases.

1. The bandage should be applied smoothly and with even tension throughout.

2. Since the plaster expands slightly on setting, it must be applied tightly enough to set snugly on the part.

3. The bandage should never be twisted during the process of application.

4. The part must be maintained and held in the desired position until the plaster is dry, otherwise the fractured bones may move out of position.

5. The assistant holding the limb must not keep the hands in one place since he may produce a depression of the plaster at one point, which may subsequently press on the skin and produce pressure sores.

6. Weak points in circular casts should be reinforced with molded splints.

Methods of Application

There are two principal methods of immobilization with plaster of Paris, namely:

The Circular Cast

In this method the extremity, or other part to be immobilized, is first covered with stockinet, one or two layers of sheet cotton are applied over the entire part, and pieces of felt are applied over the bony prominences. The plaster is then applied in a fashion similar to the application of an ordinary roller bandage; that is, with circular, spiral, recurrent, etc., turns which encircle the part. Thus, on completion, there is produced a solid, firm dressing of plaster which completely covers and immobilizes the part. This is referred to as a *plaster cast.* This is the ideal type of immobilization for major portions of the body, such as the thoracic and lumbar regions in fractures of the vertebrae; or for immobilization of the hip or femur in diseases of these parts; or for immobilization of the arm and shoulder in fractures in this region. (See Fig. 520.)

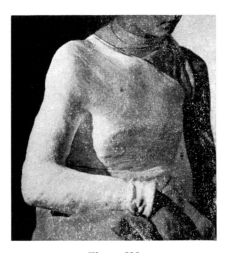

Figure 520

The circular plaster-of-Paris cast is also used for immobilization in fractures of the bones of the leg and foot. The main objection to its use here is that if any swelling takes place under the cast, an increased pressure is produced within the cast. This pressure may be sufficient to interfere with normal circulation of the part, interfering first with the venous return, and then with arterial flow. Thus, in those cases in which the plaster is applied shortly after the injury and the swelling is not very marked, special care must be taken not to apply the plaster too tightly. Although in the hands of the experienced there really is little danger following the application of circular casts, however rare as it is, circulatory embarrassment does occasionally occur, and thus special precautions must be taken to prevent this dangerous complication.

Following the application of a circular cast, the fingers or toes must be observed very carefully for any evidence of circulatory disturbance, including cyanosis, swelling, pallor, loss of sensation, and coldness. At the first appearance of any of these symptoms, the cast should be examined and cut if deemed advisable. To prevent such occurrence, many surgeons prefer to bivalve the circular casts. This consists of cutting the cast in two by making two complete cuts along the entire length of the cast, one on the medial aspect and one on the lateral aspect, or, one on the anterior and one on the posterior aspect of same. This is done shortly after the cast is applied and before it hardens fully. The cast is divided into two parts, which are then approximated and held in place by adhesive plaster strips. This method allows for slight swelling without endangering the circulation. It is advisable, particularly in those cases in which the surgeon will not have the opportunity to observe the extremity for at least 12 hours following application of the cast, to cut the circular cast. At this early stage the cast can be cut with a sharp knife or scalpel. Another advantage of the bivalved cast is that the extremity may more readily be examined from time to time, and also makes it more convenient to apply other forms of therapy, such as baking and massage, during the healing process.

Smooth casts

It is to the surgeon's advantage to apply a neat, uniformly smooth cast. To give the cast a finished appearance, the following may be done: After the completion of the cast, there is usually some plaster-of-Paris powder in the box which holds the rollers. The free plaster is mixed with water to the consistency of thick cream and is then spread smoothly over the dressing with the hands, thereby hiding the edges of the individual turns of bandage. When this has begun to set, a bright glossy surface may be given to it by rubbing with a pad of cotton saturated with alcohol.

Opening a cast "window" over a wound

Occasionally, a cast is applied over a sutured wound. From time to time it may be necessary to examine the wound long before the time for removal of the cast. In such cases a window may be made in the cast for examination of the wound. The following method has been devised for the exact localization of the site of the wound: A piece of thick lead or copper wire is molded into a ring or square, slightly larger than the size of the wound. Several layers of adhesive plaster (preferably waterproof) are wound around the wire. Before application of the plaster of Paris, the ring of wire is placed on the stockinet over the wound. The plaster is then applied around the part, incorporating the wire in the dressing. After the cast is completed, there is produced a prominence in the cast, which serves as a guide for cutting out a "window" over a wound. If the outlined square or circle is cut almost completely, leaving a small portion attached, the latter fixed part acts as a hinge for the window.

The Molded Splint

Molded splints are prepared from plaster-of-Paris roller bandages as follows: A roller is unrolled for any desired distance on a piece of flat metal or wooden board. It is then rolled back upon itself to make a double layer of plaster. This process of unrolling the plaster back and forth on itself is repeated until the layers of plaster measure about $\frac{3}{16}$ inch to $\frac{1}{4}$ inch in thickness. The plaster is then compressed and made smooth with the hands, to a homogenous splint. A piece of sheet cotton wadding, slightly longer and wider than the plaster strips, is then applied to the plaster. The sheet cotton and the plaster are then lifted off the board as a unit and applied to the part. Since the plaster is still soft, it is molded to the part. A roller gauze bandage is applied to mold the plaster firmly to the part. When dry, the plaster acts as a rigid splint, and thus is referred to as the "molded splint." (See Fig. 521.) In fractures of the forearm, particularly Colles' fracture, the molded splint is applied in a *sugar-tong* fashion. (See Fig. 522.)

Reinforcement of casts

Certain types of casts require some reinforcing, else they would readily be broken. These include hip and thigh casts and arm and shoulder casts. The body casts all require reinforcing. For this purpose, thin strips of sheet metal may be incorporated into the dressing; however, plaster-of-Paris molded splints may be used with equal effectiveness. The bandage is unrolled to the length of the desired reinforcement, and then reversed upon itself repeatedly until about 10 to 15 thicknesses of bandage are laid down as in the preparation of a molded splint, as described. This reinforcement is then applied over the weak points and incorporated into the cast with circular turns. (See Fig. 528.)

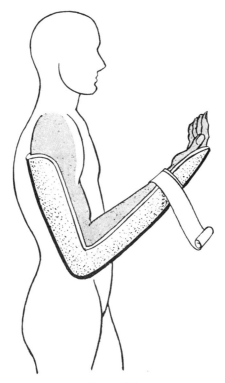

Figure 521

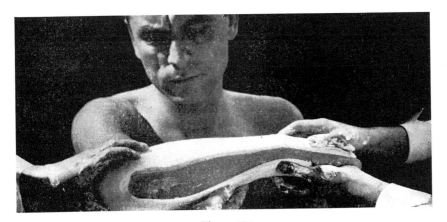

Figure 522

Maintenance of position of bone fragments

The molded splint may be of considerable value following closed reduction of fractures of the lower extremity, tibia and fibula. It is not an uncommon occurrence for the bony fragments to slip out of place while the leg is being supported and the plaster cast is being applied. In such cases, following reduction, a plaster splint is prepared and slipped under the extremity, from heel to thigh, and molded to same. When the plaster splint is dry, it serves as a rigid support which can then be used to lift the leg, without danger of displacement of the fragments. This posterior molded splint is incorporated into a circular cast which is then applied.

It is important, in the preparation of molded splints, to first measure exactly the desired length, since splints which are too long are cumbersome, and splints which are too short do not adequately serve their purpose.

7. DRYING OF PLASTER-OF-PARIS DRESSINGS

Plaster-of-Paris casts or splints may readily be cracked or broken by the patient if he moves the parts before the plaster has had the opportunity to dry sufficiently; thus, early and quick drying of the plaster is highly desirable. Most casts and splints harden shortly after application; however, full drying may not take place for 24 to 36 hours. In dry weather, the process is shorter than in damp, muggy weather. Numerous methods have been devised for hastening the drying of plaster casts. Various-sized frames, lined by electric light bulbs, may be placed over the parts. These hasten drying, but create considerable heat which may be uncomfortable for the patient. Warm-air blowers have been used over casts for hastening evaporation of the water. Probably the most practical method is to remove the bedcovers and expose the entire cast or splint to the air. A small electric light lamp, similar to those used for applying heat to various parts of the body, may be applied over the cast. This will usually prove most satisfactory.

8. REMOVAL OF PLASTER-OF-PARIS DRESSINGS

Molded splints may readily be removed by simply cutting the gauze or muslin bandages which are used to retain the splints in place. Casts, however, present a different problem. These must be cut and removed from the patient without disturbing the injured parts. The ideal method of removal is to bivalve same; that is, two cuts are made in

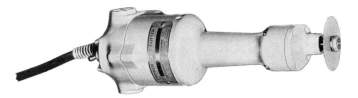

Figure 523

the cast, one on the medial aspect and one on the lateral aspect. If these are inconvenient, then anterior and posterior cuts may be made. Numerous devices are available for cutting casts. A specially constructed electric cutter makes this a simple task. (See Fig. 523.) When this is not available, other methods are used. A hand-operated cast cutter may be used. Plaster saws and plaster shears may also be utilized. (See Fig. 524.)

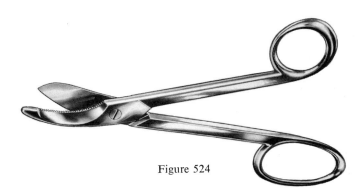

Figure 524

To facilitate the cutting of a cast, a shallow groove is made in the cast along the intended line of division. This is done with either a knife or a few strokes of the saw. Hydrogen peroxide, vinegar, or dilute hydrochloric acid is then applied along the groove with a medicine dropper. This softens the plaster so that it can be cut easily with the cutter, knife, or saw. Application of the acid or peroxide may be repeated as often as necessary until the cast is cut.

9. THE "SOFT" CAST

In certain conditions, such as chronic ulcers of the legs due to varicose veins or swelling of the legs following phlebitis, it is desirable to apply firm, even pressure over the legs for prolonged periods of time. At the same time, there is to be only partial or limited immobilization of the part. A most popular dressing for this purpose has been the *Unna paste boot,* a "soft" cast constructed of several layers of gauze bandage alternating with a paste made up of zinc oxide, gelatin, glycerin, and water. The leg is first painted with the paste. A layer of gauze bandage is then applied. This is then followed by successive layers of paste and bandage, until three or four layers of gauze have been applied. Several strips of adhesive plaster are applied over the final layer of gauze. A completely prepared Unna paste boot, ready for direct application, is now available commercially as Gelocast® or Cruricast®. Because of ease of application and effectiveness in maintaining partial immobilization, these are used for a variety of purposes, including strains and sprains of the ankles, as well as a first dressing after the removal of a rigid cast which has been in place for a number of weeks for the treatment of a fracture.

UNIT EIGHT ...

COSMETIC BANDAGING AND DRESSING

"In the application of the dressing we must not sacrifice the useful to the agreeable; but, if it be possible to give some elegance to the bandage, while we have made it at the same time better, why should we not do so?"

Alf. A. L. M. Velpeau

28

Cosmetic Bandaging

1. Introduction.
2. Cosmetic bandaging, defined.
3. Cosmetic bandaging materials.
4. Cosmetic bandaging technics.

1. INTRODUCTION

Heretofore, we have been concerned with the presentation of basic, simplified, easily adaptable methods of bandaging, or immobilizing the various regions and parts of the body. A working knowledge of the functional method of bandaging makes it possible for one to meet almost any problem in bandaging. Occasionally, however, there arises the necessity for deviation from basic principles and modification of the standard systems. This is usually in response to the desire, or demand, for inconspicuous dressings. Persons whose daily occupations bring them into frequent contact with others usually prefer to direct as little attention as possible to a site of injury, or surgical dressing.

Thus, from time to time, various physicians, nurses, and others concerned with surgical dressings, have devised ingenious methods for bandaging certain areas with relatively inconspicuous dressings. Many of these even have certain advantages over the standard methods of dressing various parts. Not only has there been modification of the technics employed, but there has also been an attempt on the part of surgical supply organizations to produce materials of such color and texture as will make the dressings further inconspicuous.

2. COSMETIC BANDAGING DEFINED

"Cosmetic bandaging" may be defined as a form of bandaging in which there is a modification of either: (a) standard principles of bandaging, or (b) standard materials for bandaging, or both, for the purpose of producing small, inconspicuous dressings of injured parts. It must be remembered, however, that at all times cosmetic bandages must fully satisfy the basic requirements of good bandaging. At no time should the comfort of the patient or the adequate functioning of the bandage be sacrificed for the purpose of producing a minimally noticeable bandage or dressing.

The purpose of this chapter will be twofold: (a) to present a review of some of the commercial products which have been introduced for cosmetic bandaging, and (b) to present various suggestions and modifications of basic bandaging as will lead to the same goal.

It is interesting to note that in many instances commercial products have been produced for the purposes of both economy and convenience in addition to the desired cosmetic effect.

3. COSMETIC BANDAGING MATERIALS

The commonly used white gauze, white muslin, white adhesive plaster, and white elastic webbing usually stand out in contrast to the color of the surrounding skin. To lessen the contrast between skin and white dressing, various pink and tan colored materials have been prepared. These include gauze, adhesive plaster, and elastic webbing.

Self-Adherent Gauze Bandage

This is a form of ordinary gauze bandage, the meshes of which are filled with a sticky substance which causes surfaces of the gauze to adhere to each other when apposed. Commercially prepared under the names of Gauztex® and Stixon®, this type of gauze is specially recommended for wounds over the fingers and toes since it obviates the necessity for any other type of fixation. Since the gauze adheres to itself, there is no slipping of one turn of gauze upon the next, and thus this material may also be used for the support of strained and sprained fingers and extremities. Applied in several layers to a finger, not only does it protect the finger but it acts almost as a splint to support and limit the motion of the part.

The gauze does not adhere to hair, skin, or clothing, nor does it loosen in water, oil, or other liquids.

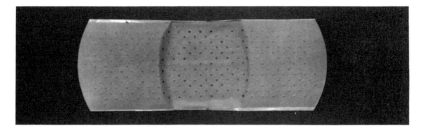

Figure 525

Ready-Prepared Adhesive-Gauze Dressings

One of the most widely used dressing for minor cuts, bruises, and abrasions is the Band-Aid®. This dressing combines a sterile gauze pad for dressing the injured part and a strip of adhesive plaster for holding the dressing in place. It is often used on the hands and fingers, the neck and face, and the feet and the toes. These vary in width from ½ inch to 6 inches, and may then be cut to any desired width. (See Figs. 525, 526.) Many of these are prepared with waterproof adhesive plaster or plastic strips. The colors are either white or pink. These dressings are packed in small individual paper envelopes which are sterilized after packing. The envelope is kept sealed until ready for use. For further cosmetic effect, and to dress very small wounds, a variety of specially-shaped and smaller Band-Aids have been produced. (See Fig. 527.)

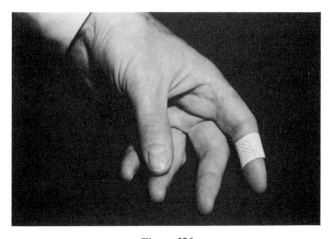

Figure 526

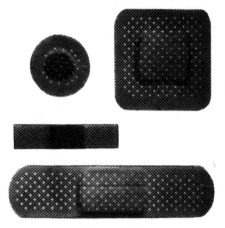

Figure 527

Ready-Prepared Plaster-of-Paris Splints

As described in an earlier chapter, molded plaster-of-Paris splints are prepared by unrolling the plaster roller and folding the material upon itself a number of times, before application. To obviate the necessity for unrolling the material, ready-cut lengths of plaster-of-Paris bandage have been commercially prepared, thereby simplifying the splint-making technic. These splints are supplied in various sizes and may be cut to any desired size or shape, before saturating with water and applying. These may be used for either reinforcing casts or for the preparation of individual splints. Several thicknesses are simply placed together, immersed in water, and then applied as a unit. (See Fig. 528.)

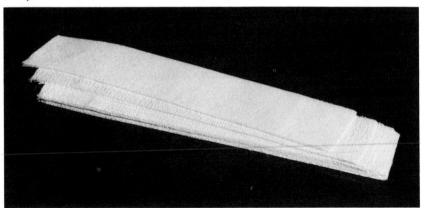

Figure 528

Plastic Splints

In response to the demand for neat, clean, lightweight, easily molded splints, a variety of these have been prepared of a crystal-clear, plastic material which is permeable to X-rays. Supplied in various sizes, the splints are immersed in hot or boiling water for a short time, and then molded to the part in the same fashion as are plaster-of-Paris molded splints. A thin layer of gauze or other padding is then applied between the skin and the splint.

Shoes for Bandaged, Taped, and Splinted Feet

Often following the application of bandages, or adhesive plaster supports to the foot, the shoe cannot be worn, and thus it becomes necessary to prepare some makeshift protection for the foot. This is usually done by cutting some old pair of shoes or slippers to accommodate the foot with its dressing. Occasionally, a patient with a plaster-of-Paris cast of the lower extremity is allowed out of bed on crutches and similar protection is prepared for the foot.

A variety of special shoes, or cast boots, have been devised for this purpose. The upper portion is made of either fabric or leather-like plastic material. The sole is either leather or plastic, and is cushioned with a thick layer of foam rubber. These are made to fit either the right or left foot, and are held securely by lacing. These shoes or boots afford protection and at the same time are neat in appearance. The Bronson® boot (See Fig. 529) and Mollo-Pedic® shoe (See Fig. 530) are two of the most commonly used boots for this purpose.

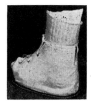

Figure 529

4. COSMETIC BANDAGING TECHNICS

Although the greater part of cosmetic bandaging is the result of the various specially prepared materials already presented, there are several modifications of technics which make for neat, less conspicuous dressings. Most of these have been directed toward bandaging of the fingers.

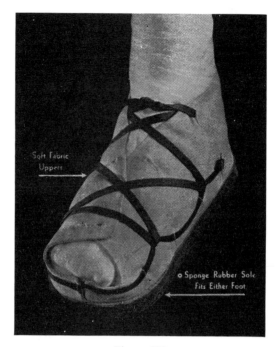

Figure 530

Maltese Cross Dressing for Fingertip

In injuries over the tip of the finger, a gauze pad is usually folded over the tip and then maintained in place by the usual turns, utilized in covering a finger. The commonly used square gauze pad, when folded over the fingertip, tends to produce a rather bulky bandage, due to the excess bulk of gauze proximal to the tip.

To eliminate this excessive bulkiness, the square gauze pad is cut to the shape of a Maltese cross. (See Figs. 531, 532.) When this is applied, no excess bulk results for the ends of the cross overlap and adapt themselves to the surface beneath. (See Fig. 533.) Having covered the tip with the cross, it is necessary merely to apply a circular strip of adhesive plaster around the base of the terminal phalanx to hold the gauze cross in place, or, the finger may then be bandaged in the usual manner, with recurrent turns over the gauze pad.

The Maltese cross may also be used for covering amputation stumps. (See Fig. 534.)

Bandaging the Finger

Bandages applied to the finger without proper anchoring at the wrist

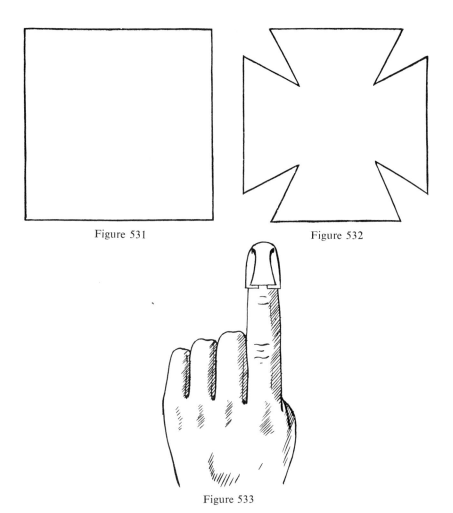

Figure 531   Figure 532

Figure 533

tend to slip off. With the proper use of adhesive plaster, the turns around
the wrist may be eliminated and the bandage applied to the finger alone.
This may be done by either one of two methods:

   Method No. 1: A piece of adhesive plaster is cut, 2 or 2½ inches
long and 1 inch wide. (See Fig. 535.)

   The adhesive is folded back upon itself in a lengthwise direction,
with the nonadherent surfaces in approximation. (See Fig. 536.)

   The adhesive strip is applied to the finger in a lengthwise manner,
on the side away from the injured area. It is so placed that one adherent surface is in contact with the finger, while the other surface faces
outward. (See Fig. 537.)

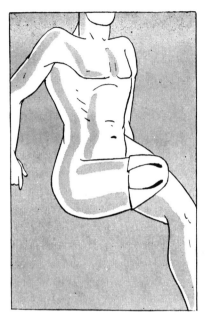

Figure 534

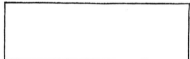

Figure 535

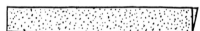

Figure 536

A series of simple spiral or spiral reverse turns is then applied to the finger, over the adhesive. The final turn is fixed with a small strip of adhesive plaster. This makes for a firm, neat bandage which will not slip off.

Method No. 2: The finger is bandaged with a one-inch bandage as follows:

(a) Apply one or two circular turns around the base of the finger;

(b) cover the tip of the finger with recurrent turns;

(c) apply spiral, or spiral reverse, turns from the tip to the base of the finger, and terminate with one or two circular turns. (See Fig. 538.)

(d) Apply two one-half-inch-wide strips of adhesive plaster as follows: Beginning on the dorsum of the base of the finger, carry the strip of adhesive over the tip and onto the palmar surface of the finger to the base of the finger. Apply a similar strip from the medial aspect of the base of the finger around the tip to the lateral aspect of the base of the finger. (See Fig. 539.)

(e) Apply two circular strips of adhesive, one at the base and one over the distal end of the finger. (See Fig. 540.)

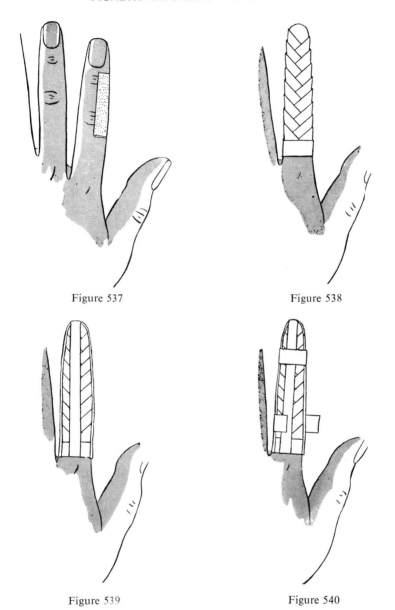

Figure 537

Figure 538

Figure 539

Figure 540

Tubular Gauze Dressings

These are specially prepared products, made of cotton which is woven into seamless, tubular rolls. These dressings are applied with special metal applicators of various sizes. Tubegauz® is particularly effective in rapid and neat bandaging of fingers, hands, feet, and toes.

UNIT NINE ...

A PRACTICAL METHOD
OF PRESENTING BANDAGING

Among the Hindus five to ten centuries before Christ, surgical treatment attained a high point of development. Their manuscripts describe a variety of surgical instruments and important procedures. They devised the bamboo splint centuries afterward adopted by the British Army. They were skilled in the use of bandages, and *taught the art of bandaging by applying them to plants, fruits, stuffed leather bags and even dead animals. The student, at least, went through the motions.*

29

A Practical Method of Presenting Bandaging

1. Introduction.
2. The practice room.
3. Plan of study.
4. Examination.

1. INTRODUCTION

"Practice makes perfect" is a maxim that holds true for bandaging as well as for any other field of endeavor. Practice in bandaging, however, is limited by the fact that the student must have a subject upon whom to practice. This is usually arranged by having students learn in organized groups or classes, two students working together and alternating upon each other. Unfortunately, the time allotted to such organized practice is not very great and thus the opportunities for practice in medical schools, nurses' training schools, and Army, Navy, and Air Corps medical corps schools are grossly inadequate. A method is herein presented, which, it is believed, will make it possible for students to spend more time in the practice of bandaging.

Having learned the basic principles of bandaging, which are dependent upon a knowledge of the geometric figures of the body, and the basic turns which are applicable to these figures, the student is then ready for the *Practice Room*. A series of geometric figures and roller bandages is made available to the student, who then applies the various turns to the fundamental figures. Having mastered the basic turns with ease and dexterity, the student finds it a simple transition from these figures to the human body.

The remainder of this section will be devoted to a description and method of preparation of such a practice room, as well as the means of its utilization. It is understood, of course, that many modifications will be made of the plan herein presented; however, it is hoped that the following will serve as a guide in constructing and arranging for the practice room and its use.

2. THE PRACTICE ROOM

Location

Centrally located rooms, easily accessible from the living quarters of nurses, internes, medical students, Army, Navy, and Air Force medical corps men, would be the ideal choice from the viewpoint of location. A conveniently located room is much more conducive to study than is one which entails much inconvenience to reach.

Size

The practice room should be large enough to accommodate several persons comfortably. The size will undoubtedly vary with the availability of space; however, a minimum size of ten feet square is recommended.

Illumination

The room should be well illuminated, should have dignity and importance, and, at the same time, should be a desirable, welcome place for the bandager to spend available spare time.

Worktable

A "worktable," about 30 inches above the floor and about 15 inches wide, should be built against the wall, all around the room. Comfortable chairs should be available but the use of these should not be encouraged since the bandager is usually standing when applying a bandage.

Figures and Models

These consist of the three basic figures described earlier in the book and are: (a) cylinders; (b) truncated cones, and (c) ovoids.

These figures may be made in their natural size as found in the body and may be constructed of a variety of materials. Wood or various plastic materials may be used, and then these may be covered with collodion to prevent excessive slipping of the bandage. Stockinet, such as is used beneath plaster-of-Paris casts, makes a fine covering material. As an alternate suggestion, the same type of stockinet may be used to prepare the various figures and then these may be filled with some soft material, or sand, in the same manner as the soft, flexible dolls are prepared. These figures are then mounted on individual bases.

Additional figures may be added later, depending upon the availability of materials. These would include models of the hand, foot, lower abdomen and thighs, and the shoulder, chest, and arm.

Several of each of the basic figures should be available. These are then set at even distances apart on the worktable.

Bandaging Materials

Muslin is the material of choice for the practice of bandaging since it is firm, durable, easily laundered, and requires the most care and accuracy in the preparation of a good bandage. Various widths of muslin should be available. These include: 1, 2, 3, and 4 inch.

A rolling machine should be available so that, after using a bandage, the student can reroll it and leave it ready for use by the next student. A small cabinet is provided for the storage of these rollers of bandage. From time to time, these rolls should be laundered to maintain the tidiness of the practice room.

Clock

A large clock with a second hand should be suspended on the wall so that the student may time himself or herself and thus determine whether or not he or she is gaining speed in bandaging.

Charts

Numerous charts should be prepared and hung in the room. These should include: (a) a large chart of the *Geometric Man,* shown earlier in the book, and demonstrating the configuration of the human body as seen by the functional bandager; (b) illustrations of the basic turns and their application to various parts of the body. Each of these should be suspended over the particular figure described; (c) quotes such as "Practice makes perfect"; axioms and truisms of bandaging.

Register

Students should register and state the time of arrival and leaving so as to determine the total time spent in the practice of bandaging.

3. PLAN OF STUDY

Introduction

The bandager should first learn to apply the basic turns to the three simple figures. He is advised to spend frequent available quarter-hours, half-hours, and even hour-periods practicing the various types of bandages. During each visit to the practice room, he should choose one figure and concentrate on same, first studying the descriptive chart, and then applying the basic turns. Having learned correct and exact application of the bandage, the bandager then strives to attain speed. When he has mastered a particular turn on a basic figure, he should then apply same to a corresponding part on the human body. Where formal courses are given in bandaging, as in nurses' training schools, etc., the greater part of the classroom work and group sessions may then consist of the application of these turns by the students upon each other, with criticism and correction of same by the instructor. This obviates the necessity for much lecturing and demonstration.

Experience Sheets

Each student should have an experience sheet upon which may be tabulated the time spent in the practice room and the various turns practiced. Thus, it is possible to obtain a good idea as to which turns have been overlooked.

A minimum number of practice room hours may be a basic requirement in a course in bandaging.

4. EXAMINATION

At the completion of the course, practical examinations are conducted, covering the application of the basic turns to the basic figures, and the further application of these principles to bandaging the human body.

UNIT TEN . . .

BIBLIOGRAPHY

30

Bibliography

ADAMS, FRANCIS: *The Genuine Works of Hippocrates,* translated from the Greek, Vol. I and II. William Wood and Company, New York, 1886.

AMERICAN MEDICAL ASSOCIATION, COMMITTEE ON FRACTURES: *Primer on Fractures,* Chicago, 1963.

AMERICAN RED CROSS: *First Aid Textbook.* The Blakiston Company, Philadelphia, Pa.

BABCOCK, W. WAYNE: *A Textbook of Surgery,* 2nd Ed. W. B. Saunders Company, Philadelphia, Pa., 1935.

BAILEY, HAMILTON: *Emergency Surgery,* 7th Ed. The Williams & Wilkins Company, Baltimore, Md., 1958.

———: *Surgery of Modern Warfare,* 2 Volumes. The Williams & Wilkins Company, Baltimore, Md., 1941.

BEEKMAN, FENWICK: *Office Surgery.* J. B. Lippincott Company, Philadelphia, Pa., 1932.

BELILIOS, A. D. AND MULVANY, D. K.: *A Handbook of First Aid Bandaging,* 4th Ed. London, 1955.

CALDWELL, JOHN A.: *A Manual of the Treatment of Fractures.* Charles C. Thomas, Springfield, Ill., 1941.

CHRISTOPHER, FREDERICK: *Minor Surgery,* 8th Ed. Edited by Alton Ochsner and Michael E. DeBakey. W. B. Saunders Co., 1959.

———: *Textbook of Surgery,* 8th Ed. Edited by Loyal Davis. W. B. Saunders Co., Philadelphia, Pa., 1964.

COLE, WARREN H.: *Textbook of Surgery,* 7th Ed. Appleton-Century-Crofts, New York, 1959.

——— AND PUESTOW, CHARLES H.: *First Aid, Diagnosis and Management,* 6th Ed. Appleton-Century-Crofts, New York, 1965.

CONWELL, H. EARLE AND REYNOLDS, FRED C.: *Key and Conwell's Management of Fractures, Dislocation, and Sprains,* 7th Ed. Mosby & Co., St. Louis, 1961.

COPE, ZACHARY: *Some Principles of Minor Surgery.* Oxford University Press, New York, 1929.

288

COTTON, FREDERIC J.: *Dislocations and Joint Fractures,* 2nd Ed. W. B. Saunders Co., Philadelphia, Pa., 1924.

DESAULT, P. J.: *A Treatise on Fractures, Luxations, and Other Affections of the Bones.* Fry & Kammerer, Philadelphia, Pa., 1805.

ELIASON, ELDRIDGE L.: *First Aid in Emergencies,* 10th Ed. J. B. Lippincott Company, Philadelphia, Pa., 1941.

————: *Practical Bandaging, Including Adhesive and Plaster-of-Paris Dressings,* 5th Ed. J. B. Lippincott Company, Philadelphia, Pa., 1938.

FERGUSON, L. KRAEER AND SHOLTIS, LILLIAN A.: *Eliason's Surgical Nursing,* 11th Ed. J. B. Lippincott Company, Philadelphia, Pa., 1959.

FOOTE, EDWARD M. AND LIVINGSTON, EDWARD M.: *Principles and Practices of Minor Surgery,* 6th Ed. D. Appleton and Company, New York, 1929.

GARRISON, FIELDING H.: *An Introduction to the History of Medicine,* 4th Ed. W. B. Saunders Company, Philadelphia, Pa., 1929.

GECKELER, EDWIN O.: *Plaster of Paris Technic.* Williams and Company, Baltimore, Md., 1944.

GIBB, W. TRAVIS: *Minor Surgery in General Practice.* Paul B. Hoeber, Inc., New York, 1934.

GIBNEY, V. P.: *Sprained Ankle,* New York Medical Journal, 61: 193 (Feb., 16th) 1895.

GROLNICK, MAX: *Factors Involved in the Production of Adhesive Plaster Irritation,* American Journal of Surgery, 50: 1 (Oct.) 63, 1940.

HOERR, NORMAN L. AND OSOL, ARTHUR: *New Gould's Medical Dictionary,* 2nd Ed. The Blakiston Company, New York, 1956.

HOPKINS, WILLIAM BARTON: *The Roller Bandage,* Lippincott's Nursing Manuals. J. B. Lippincott Company, Philadelphia, Pa., 1911.

IVY, ROBERT H. AND CURTIS, LAWRENCE: *Fractures of the Jaws,* 2nd Ed., revised. Lea & Febiger, Philadelphia, Pa., 1938.

JOHNSON AND JOHNSON, INC.: *Therapeutic Uses of Adhesive Tape.* New Brunswick, N. J., 1958.

JONES, COLONEL SIR ROBERT: *Injuries to Joints.* Oxford University Press, New York, 1918.

LEWIS, KENNETH M.: *Fractures and Dislocations.* Oxford Medical Series. Oxford University Press, New York, 1941.

LIVINGSTON, EDWARD M.: *Bandaging,* Cyclopedia of Medicine, Surgery, and Specialties, Vol. II, pp. 115-149. F. A. Davis Company, Philadelphia, Pa., 1939.

————: *A Modification of the Odén Bandage for the Thorax,* J.A.M.A., 78: 429 (Feb.) 1922.

MITCHINER, PHILIP H. AND COWELL, E. M.: *Medical Organization and Surgical Practice in Air Raids,* 2nd Ed. The Blakiston Company, Philadelphia, Pa., 1941.

NEALON, THOMAS F., JR.: *Fundamental Skills in Surgery.* W. B. Saunders Co., Philadelphia, Pa., London, 1962.

OAKES, LOIS: *Illustrations of Bandaging and First Aid,* 4th Ed. The Williams & Wilkins Company, Baltimore, Md., 1950.

PYE, WALTER: *Surgical Handicraft.* Edited by Hamilton Bailey; 17th Ed. The Williams & Wilkins Company, Baltimore, Md., 1956.

RAWLING, L. BATHE: *Landmarks and Surface Markings of the Human Body.* Paul B. Hoeber, Inc., New York, 1911.

RING, P. A.: *The Care of the Injured.* E. & L. Livingstone, Ltd., Edinburgh and London, 1964.

ROBINSON, VICTOR: *The Story of Medicine.* Tudor Publishing Company, New York, 1936.

ROMANIS, WILLIAM H. C. AND MITCHINER, PHILIP H.: *The Science and Practice of Surgery,* 3rd Ed. William Wood and Company, New York, 1930.

SCUDDER, CHARLES LOCKE: *The Treatment of Fractures,* 11th Ed., revised. W. B. Saunders Company, Philadelphia, Pa., 1938.

THORNDIKE, AUGUSTUS: *A Manual of Bandaging, Strapping, and Splinting,* 3rd Ed. Lea & Febiger, Philadelphia, Pa., 1959.

TRUMBLE, HUGH: *Made-to-Order Splints: The Technique of Construction and Field of Application.* British Journal of Surgery, 19: 292 (Oct.) 1931.

VELPEAU, ALF. A. L. M.: *New Elements of Operative Surgery, Augmented with a Treatise on Minor Surgery,* Vol. I. Samuel S. & William Wood, New York, 1847.

WHARTON, HENRY R.: *Minor and Operative Surgery, Including Bandaging.* Lea & Febiger, Philadelphia, Pa., 1913.

WHITING, A. D.: *Bandaging,* 3rd Ed., revised. W. B. Saunders Company, Philadelphia, Pa., 1929.

Index

Abdomen, bandage for, 124
Absorbent cotton, 17
  preparation of, 17
  uses of, 17
Ace bandage, 22
Adaptic bandage®, 22
Adhesive "butterfly" in small wounds, 201
Adhesive plaster, 17
  as substitute for sutures, 201, 202
  binders, 197
  butterfly, 201
  corsets, 197
  fixation of dressings, 195
    large wounds, 196
    small wounds, 195
  for epithelialization of wounds, 218
  immobilization, 205
    of ankle, 205
    of back, 212
    of chest, 214
    of knee, 207
  in bivalved casts, 217
  in large, unsutured wounds, 202
  non-irritating types of, 193
    Dermicel®, 193
    Micropore®, 193
  preparation of, 17
  preparation of skin for, 193
  principles of application, 193
  removal of, 218
  skin preparation for, 193
    Ace Adherent®, 194
    Aeroplast®, 194
    collodion, 194
    Mercurochrome®, 194
    tincture of benzoin, 194
  skin reaction to, 193
  starting of bandages, 195
  terminating of bandages, 195
  traction in fractures, 217
  types of, 192
    regular, 192
    special strapping, 193
    waterproof, 193
  uses of, 19, 192
Airplane splint for humerus, 231
Amputation stump, bandage for, 183, 274
Ankle, bandaging of, 97
  taping the, 205
Arm, bandaging of, 82
  triangle for, 173
Arteries of leg, 94
Axioms of good bandaging, 54

Back strapping, 212

Band-Aids®, 271
Bandage, 8
  Ace®, 22
  Adaptic®, 22
  Barton, 116
  capeline, of head, 113
  compound, 8
  compression, 18
  cravat, 8, 157
  demi-gauntlet, 70
  gauntlet, 79
  good, requirements of, 7
  handkerchief, 9
  immobilization, 10
  immovable, 10
  Livingston, 143
  movable, 10
  Peg®, 23
  roller, 11
  Scultetus, 11, 126
  simple, 12
  spica, defined, 12
  triangle, defined, 15
    fixation of, 159
    "Functional" approach to, 158
    parts of, 158
    preparation of, 155
  Velpeau, 138, 139
Bandager, defined, 8
Bandages, anatomico-physiological application of, 63
  fixation of, 48
    adhesive plaster, 48
    circular, 48
    oblique, 48
  functions of, 6
  purposes of, 6
  spica, 47
  starting of, 48, 195
  tailed, 13
    double-T, 13
    four-tailed, 14
    many-tailed, 15
    T-, 13
  termination of, 49, 195
    folding, 52
    sewing, 52
    typing with roller, 51
    with adhesive plaster, 51
    with safety pin, 52
Bandaging, cosmetic, defined, 270
Bandaging, "Functional", 6
Bandaging the abdomen, 124
  the ankle, 97
  the arm, 82
  the breast, shoulder, and thorax, 130

the breasts, 133, 134
the buttocks and thigh, 150
the chest, 122
the elbow, 83
the eye, 113
the eyes, 114
the fingers, 74, 79
the foot, 96
the forearm, 81
the groin and thigh, 147
the groins, 149
the heel, 99
the knee, 102
the leg, 91, 102
the mastoids, 115
the neck, 109, 117
the neck and axilla, 118
the neck and axillae, 119
the neck and chest, 119
the neck and head, 110
the palm and dorsum of the hand, 66
the perineum, 151
the scalp, 112
the shoulder, 136, 143
the thigh, 105
the thumb, 79
the toes, 91
the wrist, 66
Bandagist, defined, 8
Barton bandage, 116
"Baseball finger", splint for, 236
Bass-wood splints, 249
Bellevue tie, for bandages, 51
Binder, defined, 8
    double-T, for breasts, 134
    four-tailed, for jaw, 116
    many-tailed, 126
Breast, bandage for, 130
Breasts, binder for, 133, 134
Bronson Boot®, 273

Capeline bandage of head, 113
Cast, "window" in, 261
Cast, soft, 265
    Cruricast®, 266
    Gelocast®, 266
Casts, bivalving of, 261
    cutting of, 264
    reinforcement of, 262
    removal of, 264
    smooth, 261
Cellulose, 18
Cervical brace, 241
Chest, bandage for, 122
    strapping of, 214
    triangle for, 176
Circular cast, 259
Circular turns, 29
    directions for, 29
    uses of, 31
Clavicle, fracture of, 229
    anatomy of, 229
    principles of treatment, 229
    triangle for, 169
Clavicular cross, 229

Coaptation splint, 249
Colles' fractures, 233
    anatomy of, 233
    principles of treatment, 233
Collins' hitch for traction, 247
Combines, dressing, 18
    preparation of, 18
    uses of, 18
Compound bandage, 8
Cones, bandaging of, 33
Cosmetic bandaging, defined, 270
    materials for, 270
        adhesive-gauze dressings, 271
        Bronson Boot®, 273
        flesh-colored materials, 270
        Mollo-pedic® shoes, 273
        plastic splints, 273
        prepared plaster splints, 272
        self-adherent gauze, 270
Cotton, absorbent, 17
    non-absorbent, 22
    wadding, 18
Cravat bandage, 8, 157
    for hand, 183
    for temple, forehead, and chin, 167
Crepitus in fractures, 224
Crinoline, 18
"Cross-taping", 196
Cruricast®, 266
Cylinders, bandaging of, 29

Demi-gauntlet bandage, 70
Dermicel®, 193
Dislocation, defined, 8
Double-roller bandage, 11
Dressing combines, 18

Elbow, bandage for, 83
    fracture of, 232
        anatomy of, 232
        principles of treatment of, 232
Emergency splinting, 245
Eye bandage, 113
Eyes, bandages for, 114

Felt, 18
Femur, fractures of, 237
    anatomy of, 237
    principles of treatment, 237
Figure-of-eight, 43
    of ankle, 97
    of elbow, 83
    of foot, 97
    of head and neck, 111
    of knee, 102
    of neck and axilla, 118
    of neck and chest, 119
    of palm and wrist, 67
Figure-of-eight turns, 43
    classification of, 43
        ascending, 45
        converging or concentric, 45
        descending, 45
        diverging or eccentric, 45
    directions for application, 43
    uses of, 47

Fingers, bandaging of, 74, 79
  cosmetic bandages for, 274, 275
Finger-tip, bandaging of, 76
Fixed traction, 245, 246
Flannel, 18
Foam rubber, 19
Foot, bandaging of, 96
  triangle for, 180
Forearm, bandaging of, 81
Forehead, triangle for, 167
Fracture, 9, 224
  Colles', 233
  compound, 9, 224
  emergency management of, 244
    bleeding, 244
    compound wound, 244
    shock, 244
    splinting, 245
  signs and symptoms of, 224
  simple, 9, 224
Fractures of clavicle, 229
  of elbow, 232
  of femur, 237
  of humerus, 230
  of leg and ankle, 238
  of metacarpals, 233
  of phalanges, 236
  of radius, 233
  of vertebrae, 240
Functional bandaging, 6
Furacin® gauze, 22

Gauntlet bandage, 79
Gauze, 19
  grading of, 19
  self-adherent, 270
  sponges; 20
  uses of, 19, 20
Gauztex®, 270
Gelocast®, 266
Geometric configuration of body, 5
Gibney strapping for ankle, 205
Groin and thigh, bandage for, 147

Hand, cravat for, 183
  triangle for, 173
Handkerchief bandage, 9
"Hatch-taping", 196
Heel, bandage for, 99
Hip, triangle for, 179
Humerus, fracture of, 230
  anatomy of, 230, 231
  principles of treatment, 231
Hyperextension in spine injuries, 250

Immobilization, 254
  bandage, 10
  materials for, 254
    characteristids of, 254
    classification of, 254
Immovable bandage, 10

Jaw, bandage for, 116
Jones splint for humerus, 232
Keller-Blake splint, 245

Kling®, 20
Knee, bandage for, 102
  triangle for, 179
Knee-taping, 207
Knot, square or reef, 159

Leg, bandage for, 91, 102
  fractures of, 238
"Line-taping", 196
Livingston's bandage for shoulder
  and thorax, 143
Lymphatics, superficial, 62

Maltese cross dressing, 274
  for amputation stump, 274
  for finger tip, 274
Mastoid, bandage for, 115
Metacarpals, fractures of, 233
Microdon®, 22
Molded splints, 262
  preparation of, 262
  reinforcement of casts with, 262
  temporary immobilization with, 264
Mollo-pedic® shoes, 273
Montgomery tapes, 200
Movable bandage, 10
Muscles of arm, 67
  of forearm, 67, 68
  of leg, 92
  of thigh, 93
Muslin, uses of, 20

Neck and axilla, bandage for, 118
  double spica, for, 119
Neck and chest, bandage for, 119
Neck and head, bandage for, 110
Neck, bandage for, 109, 117
Nerves, superficial, 61, 63
Non-absorbent cotton, uses of, 22
Non-adhesive dressings, 22
  Adaptic®, 22
  Furacin® gauze, 22
  Microdon®, 22
  Telfa®, 22
  Vaseline® gauze, 22

Ovoids, bandaging of, 39

"Package turns" for head, 109
Peg® bandage, 23
Perineum, T-binder for, 157
Phalanges, fractures of, 236
Pillow splint for ankle, 250
Plan of study for bandaging, 281
Plaster, adhesive, 17
Plaster of Paris, 255
  bandages, 255
  care of, 255
  casts, 259
  chemistry of, 255
  drying of, 264
  manipulation of, 257
    care of hands, 257
    dipping of plaster, 257

removal from water and compression, 258
preparation for use of, 255
  patient, 256
  room and bed, 256
removal of, 264
types of, 255
  average setting, 255
  rapid setting, 255
  slow setting, 255
Plastic splints, 273
Practice room for bandaging, 282
Pronation, defined, 11

Recurrent turns, 39
  directions for, 40
  uses of, 42
Roller bandage, 11
Roller, double, 11
Rubber bandages, 21
  foam, 19
Russell's traction, 238

Scalp, bandage for, 112
  triangle for, 165
Scapula, triangle for, 171
Scultetus bandage, 11, 126
Scultetus, Johannis, 126
Shock, treatment for, 244
Shoulder, bandage for, 136, 143
  triangle for, 171
Slings for hand, forearm, and arm, 161
  broad sling (high), 164
  broad sling (low), 163
  narrow sling, 163
Spanish windlass in traction, 248
Spica bandage, defined, 12, 47
Spica, double, for breasts, 133, 134
  for groins, 149
  for neck and axilla, 119
  of breasts, 130
  of buttocks, 150
  of groin, 147
  of shoulder, 136, 143
  of thumb, 79
Spine injury, lifting patient with, 250
  splinting, 250
Spiral reverse turns, 34
  classification, 37
    ascending, 37
    descending, 37
  directions for, 34
  uses of, 38
Spiral turns, 31
  classification, 32
    rapid ascending, 32
    rapid descending, 32
    slow ascending, 32
    slow descending, 32
  directions for, 31
  uses of, 32
"Splint 'em where they lie," 243
Splint, Airplane, for humerus, 231
  bass-wood, 249

coaption, 249
Keller-Blake, 245
pillow, for ankle, 250
"sugar-tong", 262
Thomas, 245, 247
walking, 240
Splinting the lower extremity, 246
  the spine, 250
  the upper extremity, 247
Splints, defined, 12, 223
  for ankle, 250
  for clavicle, 229
    clavicular cross, 229
    figure-of-eight bandage, 229
    strap, 229
  for femur, 245
  for humerus, 230, 231
    Airplane, 231
    Robert Jones, 232
  for metacarpals, 233
  for phalanges, 236
  for vertebrae, 241
    cervical brace, 241
    Taylor brace, 241
  functions of, 223
  materials used for, 226
  molded plaster, 226
  plastic, 273
  qualities of good, 226
  uses of, 223
Sprain, defined, 13
Square knot, 159
Starting of bandages, 48
Steri-Strip®, 202
Stixon®, 270
Stockinet, 22
Strain, defined, 13
Strapping, adhesive plaster, 205
  of ankle, 205
  of back, 212
  of chest, 214
  of knee, 217
Stump, amputation, triangle for, 183
Subluxation, defined, 13
"Sugar-tong" splints, 262
Supination, defined, 13
Suspensory of breast, 133

Tailed bandages, 13
  double-T, 13
  four-tailed, 14
  many-tailed, 15
  T-, 13
Taping, defined, 15
  the ankle, 205
  the back, 212
  the chest, 214
  the knee, 207
Taylor brace for spine, 241
Telfa®, 22
Terminating of bandages, 49, 195
Thigh, bandage for, 105
Thomas splint, 245, 247
Thumb, bandaging of, 79
Toes, bandaging of, 91

Traction, adhesive plaster, 217
  Russell, for femur, 238
Triangle bandage, defined, 15, 155
  fixation of, 159
  for amputation stump, 183
  for arm, 173
  for chest, 176
  for clavicle, 169
  for foot, 180
  for hand, 173
  for hip, 179
  for knee, 179
  for palm, 183
  for scalp, 165
  for scapula, 171
  for shoulder, 171
  for temple, forehead, and chin, 167
  "Functional approach" to, 158
  naming of, 160
  parts of, 150
  preparation of, 155

Turns, basic, defined, 27
  classified, 27
    circular, 29
    figure-of-eight, 43
    recurrent, 39
    spiral, 31
      types of, 32
    spiral reverse, 34
      types of, 37

Vaseline® gauze, 22
Veins, superficial, 61
Velpeau, Alfred L.M., 139
  bandage, 138
Vertebral column, fractures, 240
  anatomy, 240
  principles of treatment, 241

Walking splint, 240
Webbing, 22
Wrist, bandage for, 66